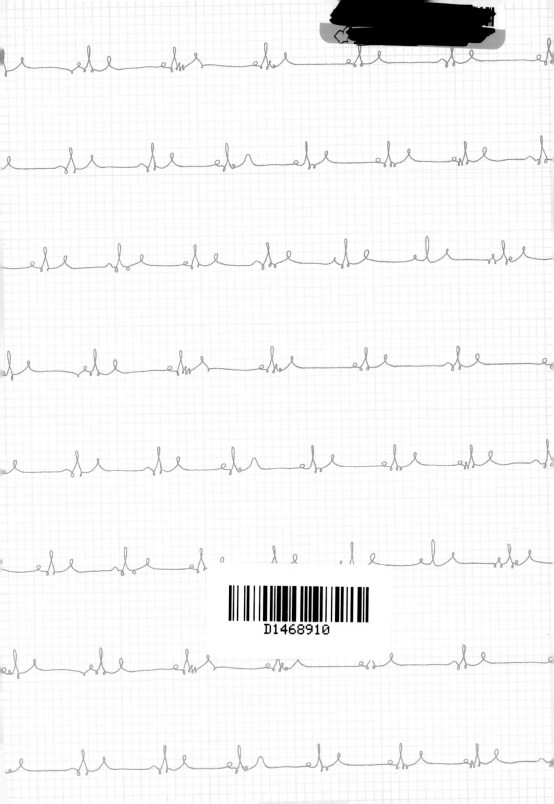

Health Design Thinking

CREATING PRODUCTS AND SERVICES FOR BETTER HEALTH

Bon Ku, MD
Ellen Lupton

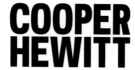

COOPER HEWITT

Published by Cooper Hewitt,
Smithsonian Design Museum
2 East 91st Street
New York, NY 10128
USA
cooperhewitt.org

Distributed by the MIT Press
Massachusetts Institute of Technology
Cambridge, Massachusetts 02142
mitpress.mit.edu

ISBN 978-0-262-53913-5

Library of Congress Control Number:
2019952263

DIRECTOR OF CROSS-PLATFORM PUBLISHING
Pamela Horn

CROSS-PLATFORM PUBLISHING ASSOCIATE
Matthew Kennedy

BOOK DESIGN Ellen Lupton

ILLUSTRATIONS Jennifer Tobias

TYPEFACES National, by Kris Sowersby,
Klim Type; Graphik, by Christian Schwartz,
Commercial Type; Edita, by Pilar Cano,
TypeTogether.

2020 2021 2022 2023 2024 / 10 9 8 7 6 5 4 3 2 1

Printed and bound in China

Smithsonian Design Museum

Contents

Principles

Methods

Case Studies

Created for design thinkers working across the health care sector, this book is illustrated with real-world challenges and compelling human stories. *Health Design Thinking* helps answer the question, How might we achieve better health through improved services, products, interactions, and education? In the United States alone, daunting challenges face the delivery of health care. Patients encounter limited access—and have difficulty navigating systems even when access is available. Clinicians feel overwhelmed and disillusioned by expanding paperwork and caseloads. Burnout among doctors is a growing crisis. Meanwhile, disparities in health outcomes are widening across communities. Health care itself has consumed 18% of the U.S. GDP and threatens to engulf ever more resources.

In the midst of these challenges, design thinking can help stakeholders create products and practices that are more humane, efficient, and equitable. *Health Design Thinking* highlights products, prototypes, and research generated by leading design firms, companies, research centers, and schools of medicine that are applying design thinking to a range of health care situations.

Authors Bon Ku and Ellen Lupton represent two institutions seeking to improve life through design thinking: Sidney Kimmel Medical College at Thomas Jefferson University, one of the oldest and largest medical schools in the U.S., and Cooper Hewitt, Smithsonian Design Museum, the only museum in the U.S. dedicated to studying the history and future of design. The Health Design Lab at Jefferson University, established in 2016, has developed an integrated longitudinal design curriculum for medical students. Cooper Hewitt is a global platform for design and a leading voice for design as a force of positive change. The museum engages designers, educators, policy makers, and citizens through exhibitions, publications, online resources, and educational outreach initiatives.

Jennifer Tobias—a gifted artist, scholar, and librarian—has graced these pages with dozens of illustrations. Pamela Horn, Cooper Hewitt's Director of Cross-Platform publishing, helped develop the concept for this book and provided expert editorial guidance from start to finish. Prominent designers, innovators, and organizations contributed case studies, including several from Maryland Institute College of Art (MICA), where Ellen Lupton serves as senior faculty.

Design challenges found in the health care space range from reducing unnecessary cesarean deliveries to reimagining hospital waiting areas and creating medical devices that enable more patients to access treatment. This book is written from inside the U.S. health care system—the most complex and cumbersome in the world. As medical systems around the globe struggle to expand access, improve outcomes, and control costs, leaders in the field of medicine are finding inspiration in health design thinking.

Cooper Hewitt, Smithsonian Design Museum is proud to collaborate with the Health Design Lab at Thomas Jefferson University to create accessible design tools for a broad audience of people engaged with the art and science of health care as a human-centered practice.

Caroline Baumann
DIRECTOR
Cooper Hewitt, Smithsonian Design Museum

Health design thinking is an approach to generating creative ideas and solutions that enhance human well-being in the context of medicine. Health design thinking is an open mindset rather than a rigid methodology. This emerging practice has been used to transform products, environments, workflows, and mission statements, and to bring new perspectives to medical professionals. Health care systems around the world employ design teams to improve patient care. Global companies embrace design thinking as a strategy for driving health care innovation. Anyone can participate in this process. Interviews, observations, storytelling, prototyping, and role-playing are tools for helping teams build empathy and address challenges.

The first section of this book explores the guiding Principles of design thinking. Next, diverse Methods explore ways to listen, observe, and make. A series of inspiring Case Studies show design in action. Each section is illustrated with research and projects from hospitals, medical schools, and communities.

Our methodology emerged from the work of the Health Design Lab at Thomas Jefferson University, founded by Bon Ku. The Lab began as an experiment. Could medical students with no engineering background create prototypes for new devices? The process works because our design teams focus on human problems, not technology. Users are included in the design proces. This educational immersion helps clinicians cultivate empathy and creativity.

Health Design Thinking applies design methods to the unique challenges of medicine. Health care should be a beautiful experience for patients, caregivers, and clinicians. We created this book for doctors, nurses, educators, students, patients, advocates, architects, and designers. Health care problems often involve ambiguity and uncertainty. Health design thinking can help us embrace the art of listening and the need to ask better questions, as we learn to value both qualitative insight and quantitative evidence.

Bon Ku, MD
ASSISTANT DEAN FOR HEALTH AND DESIGN
Sidney Kimmel Medical College at
Thomas Jefferson University

Ellen Lupton
SENIOR CURATOR, CONTEMPORARY DESIGN
Cooper Hewitt, Smithsonian Design Museum

Contributors

Dozens of clinicians, designers, patients, engineers, organizations, and advocates contributed chapters to this book. Individual images and related content are credited in the captions.

Design Process Map

PRINCIPLES Since the 1990s, thousands of groups and individuals have explored the practice of design thinking. Notable pioneers include the design consultancy IDEO and Stanford University's d.school. Design thinking has been mapped in a variety of ways—as an open spiral, a twisted loop, a double diamond, or a row of circles. Regardless of how we diagram the process, two core values or principles recur in design thinking methodologies.

First, design thinking is *human centered*. It starts with the needs and desires of people, rather than with a business proposition or an artistic idea. Human-centered design involves observation, conversation, research, and collaboration.

Second, design thinking adopts a *creative mindset*, favoring open-ended exploration over a straight path headed toward a given outcome. The creative process involves asking questions, visualizing ideas, creating tangible prototypes, and telling stories about people, ideas, and outcomes.

These core principles—human centered and creative mindset—fuel the living, changing process of design thinking. This book begins by exploring these principles in relation to examples drawn from the unique context of health care.

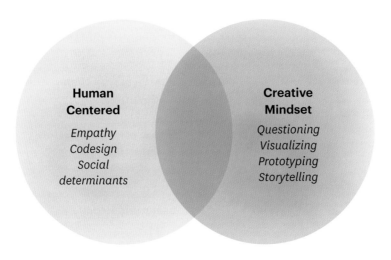

Human Centered

Empathy
Codesign
Social determinants

Creative Mindset

Questioning
Visualizing
Prototyping
Storytelling

METHODS In theory, the design process breaks down into three main phases, as shown in the diagram below. In practice, however, you can start anywhere and make your own path.

The first step is to *observe*. This requires looking, listening, asking questions, and gathering research. Observation requires patience, care, and humility. User interviews build empathy and reveal insights. Workshops facilitate codesign with diverse stakeholders. Researching the life of a community yields deeper knowledge. The values of human-centered design ground each of these methods.

The next step is to *imagine*. This involves generating multiple ideas, sorting them into groups, seeking relationships and analogies, and deciding how to move forward. Here, human-centered research mixes with creative thinking, opening our minds to unexpected concepts.

The third step is to *make*. Creative action now surges into the foreground. Making is hands-on and physical. Prototypes show how a product could work. Storyboards explain how users might interact with a device. Role-playing embodies a service or process in a social and physical way. Each creative method leads back to asking how a design solution or insight could help real people. Each prototype or narrative is a tool for communicating with users and stakeholders.

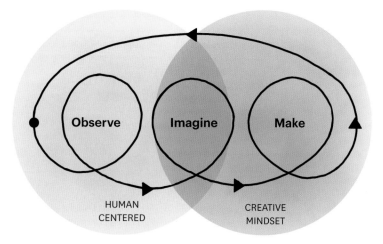

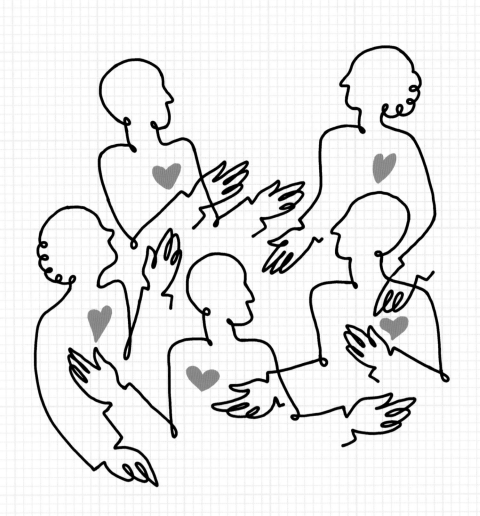

Principles

Two core principles illuminate the rich and varied practice of health design thinking. First, by embracing a human-centered perspective, each person becomes a more caring listener and a keener observer. This work requires patience and attention. Next, by actively applying a creative mindset to design and health care, we become inventors, makers, and storytellers, equipped to help build a culture of wellness. People don't think of health care as a creative field. Clinicians feel inspired when they discover that they can apply creativity to medicine.

Human Centered

Design is the ancient practice of shaping materials to achieve goals and express beliefs. Human beings and other creatures make tools and build structures in order to survive, thrive, and dominate their surroundings. Unlike other organisms, people learn from each other, creating new ideas and inventions that spread quickly.

Designers learn to look at a given situation—from the layout of a room to the shape of a door handle—and consider how it could be changed, improved, or embellished. Human-centered design asks how new approaches to a problem might improve people's lives. Well-being is the ultimate goal of any human-centered intervention.

You might be wondering, "Isn't all design human centered?" In fact, the design process doesn't always focus on the needs or desires of individuals. During the Industrial Revolution, familiar things once made by hand—from tableware to textiles—were produced with machines and sold for profit, while steam locomotives, plumbed toilets, and other new technologies transformed cities and homes around the globe. A door handle could be designed with rococo curves or cubist angles to express a unique artistic sensibility, or it could be engineered with modular parts for low-cost manufacturing.

The concept of shaping products to the human body (ergonomics) appeared in the mid-twentieth century, when designers began using research on human behavior and anatomy to simplify everything from telephones to farm equipment. Lever-style door handles—now standard in hospitals and public buildings—allow hands-free operation. This innovation, which reflects the principles of universal design, rejected the conventional pattern of the round doorknob.

More recently, users have become active participants in the design process. Human-centered design is inclusive and collaborative, approaching members of a community as experts in their own life challenges. Users are active participants and creators of knowledge, not passive subjects to be measured and manipulated.

DESIGN FOR DOOR HARDWARE
This drawing shows how designer John De Cesare applied decorative forms to hardware for a door. Functionally, the door follows the traditional form of a round doorknob, which is difficult for some people to grasp and twist. Drawing, Study 141b (detail), 1957; John De Cesare (American, b. Italy, 1890–1972); Color pencil, graphite on cream wove paper; 61.1 × 48.5 cm (24 1/16 × 19 1/8 in.); Gift of the Estate of John De Cesare, 1982-25-70; Cooper Hewitt, Smithsonian Design Museum; Photo: © Smithsonian Institution

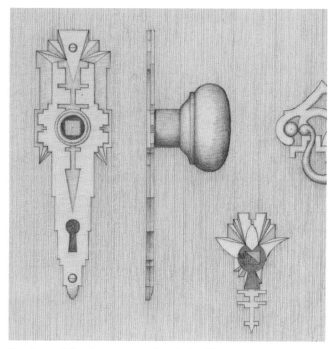

Designed for beauty and originality

LEVERON DOOR HANDLE ATTACHMENT
This plastic attachment was designed to be added to conventional round doorknobs. The lever allows a person to open the door without grasping and twisting. Such movements are difficult for people with limited hand use and for anyone carrying a package or small child. The bright color enhances visibility, making the knob easier to locate. Leveron Door Handle Attachment, 1983; Manufactured by Lindustries; H x W x D: 7.6 × 16.5 × 15.2 cm (3 × 6 1/2 × 6 in.); Gift of Lindustries; 2014-47-2; Collection of Cooper Hewitt, Smithsonian Design Museum; Photo: © Smithsonian Institution

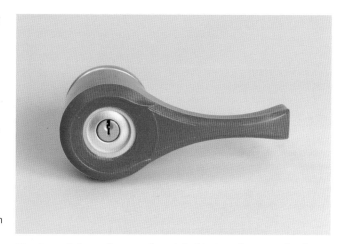

Designed for a better fit with diverse human bodies

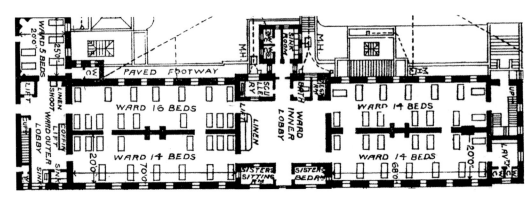

OPEN WARDS The London Hospital (1752) maximized patient density and visibility—at the expense of privacy and comfort. See John D. Thompson and Grace Goldin, *The Hospital: A Social and Architectural History* (New Haven: Yale University Press, 1975) and Jeanne Kisacky, *Rise of the Modern Hospital: An Architectural History of Health and Healing, 1870–1940* (Pittsburgh: University of Pittsburgh Press, 2017).

PATIENT-CENTERED ARCHITECTURE
This sketch of a patient room, by architect Earl S. Swensson, considers the needs of many users, including the patient, family members, nurses, and caregivers. It provides space for personal possessions, seating for visitors, and a workstation for nurses, along with an accessible bathroom. Earl Swensson Associates (ESa) designs hospitals and health care facilities. From Richard L. Miller, Earl S. Swensson, and J. Todd Robinson, *Hospital and Healthcare Facility Design*, 3rd ed. (New York: W. W. Norton, 2012). Drawing © Earl S. Swensson, FAIA Emeritus/Earl Swensson Associates

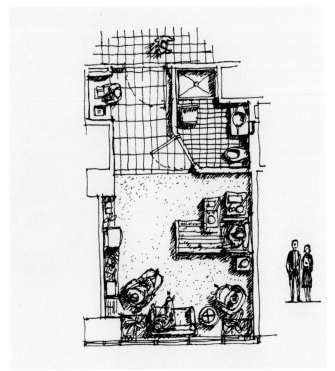

Like the design profession, the health care field has sharpened its focus on human needs. Early hospitals in the West, which belonged to churches, applied spiritual care to the ailing body. As medicine became more scientific, charitable hospitals were established to tend to the poor. The patients in these places had no power and no great chance of being healed. They were research subjects in the drive to uncover the science of disease. (Wealthy people were cared for in their private homes by doctors.)

In the early twentieth century, modern hospitals signaled the rising power of the doctor, who became one of society's most admired members. Nursing was elevated from a marginal occupation to a respected profession. Open wards were replaced with private and semiprivate rooms, attracting wealthy patients. Designed for cleanliness and efficiency, modern hospitals enabled people to recover from illness and injury in ways once unimaginable. Yet these monuments to progress could be forbidding, unwelcoming places.

Historically, hospitals have resembled anything from monasteries or a prisons to hotels or office towers. Today, vast health networks sprawl acoss cities and regions, serving as engines of employment and economic growth. Contemporary hospitals are places of constant coming and going, where outpatient treatments are more common than extended stays. Hospital design must account for complex equipment, disaster-safe infrastructure, and the daily flow of thousands of patients, families, and workers.

Doctors dominated the first modern hospitals, supported by nurses and other staff in a strict hierarchy of power and control. In the ideal hospital of today, patients occupy the center. Individuals participate in their own care and have control over their environments. Public areas and patient rooms include ample space for families, and these spaces use color, light, and materials to foster comfort.

Alas, many hospitals fail to meet these standards, and too many people lack access to care. Around the world, disparities in health outcomes reflect egregious income inequality and systemic racism. In the U.S., a patchy and opaque health care system is muddled by profit motives and political gamesmanship.

Design for health care extends beyond improving the layout of lobbies and treatment rooms and creating more ergonomic medical devices. Many opportunities for design intervention arise from the area of service design. Such projects can include anything from improving the process of obtaining informed consent to building awareness of treatments that are available but underutilized within a community. A service design project might include designing clear and engaging educational materials and developing new protocols for how clinicians exchange this information with patients and the public.

Research studies are being transformed by human-centered design, which includes stakeholders throughout the process. Medical researchers are beginning to apply design principles and methods to ask better study questions, gain fresh insight, and study the effectiveness of medical interventions. The quantitative methods of medical researchers can intersect productively with the qualitative insights of designers.

In a study of procedures for discharging pediatric patients treated with asthma in emergency departments, designers at the IIT Institute of Design collaborated with researchers at the University of Illinois at Chicago to study how people can better manage their asthma at home. Funded by a $4 million Patient-Centered Outcomes Research Institute (PCORI) grant, researchers conducted a randomized control trial called the Coordinated Healthcare Interventions for Childhood Asthma Gaps in Outcomes, or the CHICAGO Trial.

By employing the principles of codesign and prototyping, the design team created new tools aimed at improving the emergency department (ED) discharge experience. In the existing process, caregivers are subjected to a long verbal

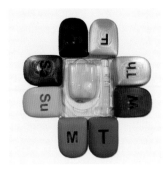

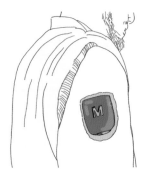

PATIENT-MADE DEVICE 3D-printed covers fit directly over an insulin pump, providing a visual reminder of when to change the injection site. Files available on Thingiverse.com.

statement accompanied by five to fifteen pages of densely typed text. The design team conducted codesign workshops with multiple stakeholders, including caregivers, primary care physicians, and ED doctors, nurses, and nurse adminstrators. They conducted interviews in family homes and observed people in six EDs. Building on this research, the team designed a new discharge tool that transforms the existing one-way, top-down information flow into a two-way conversation, organized into simple actions that can be easily implemented by clinicians. The effectiveness of this new service was compared to the usual procedure. Children whose discharge included the new patient education tool were more likely to use medications at home (including steroids, inhaler medicine, and rescue medicine) and were more likely to schedule an office visit.

The study was funded by a Patient-Centered Outcomes Research Institute (PCORI) grant, which requires patient involvement. Health design thinking challenges the current hierarchical process of medical research, which focuses on academic expertise, by actively engaging diverse stakeholders. By demonstrating the success of integrating design into research, such studies anticipate a more collaborative approach among patients, caregivers, researchers, and clinicians.

What does the future of health care hold? Medical services are moving into homes and neighborhoods. Accessible environments enable aging in place. Diagnostic tools designed for use at home allow people to monitor their heart rate,

oxygen levels, and other health indicators, and to share data with doctors. Patients are pioneering the invention of new devices and services. The Nightscout Foundation, established by families of children with diabetes, hacks existing technology so that parents can monitor glucose levels when their children are away or at school.

Diagnostic devices using mobiles phones as monitors are being deployed in communities where radiologists are in short supply. AI (artificial intelligence) systems can read such scans for early signs of cancer or diabetic blindness. Designed for use by community health workers and patients, such tools can put expertise into more hands.

Design cannot solve every health care problem. However, human-centered thinking has the power to start chipping away at entrenched patterns within the medical community and in society at large that perpetuate health inequality. Change is difficult in a hospital, where mistakes are costly and can seriously damage human lives. Not every proposal is implemented, and not every intervention succeeds. Change requires the space and the courage to test new ideas. Human-centered design is one crucial tool for distributing medical advances to more communities, not just to the most privileged. Human-centered health care sees people not as patients defined by illness or impairment but as individuals on the journey of life.

READ MORE → id.iit.edu/projects/bridging-the-communication-gap-healthcare-service-design-for-asthma-patients/; → www.pcori.org/research-results/2013/comparing-three-ways-prepare-children-and-caregivers-manage-asthma-after

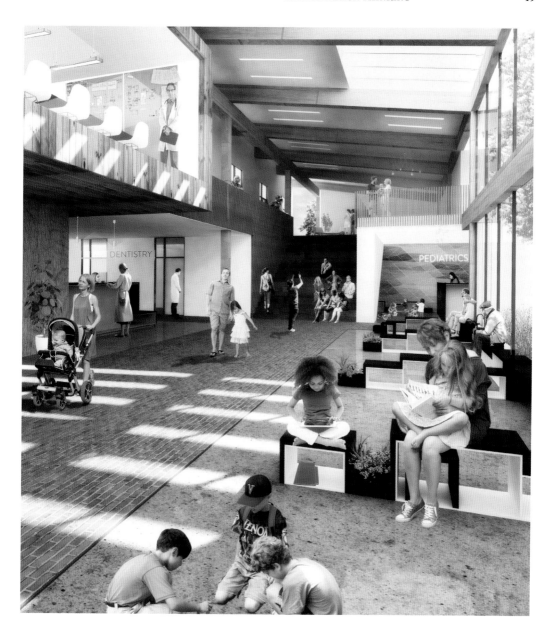

FAMILY HEALTH CENTER AT VIRGINIA PARKWAY
This patient-centered medical home is located in McKinney, Texas, a rapidly growing community where many residents lack access to primary health care and transportation services. In this new facility, primary medical, behavioral, and dental care services are integrated across a series of buildings that are united by shared social spaces. The complex is designed to serve as a dynamic community hub focused on promoting health and well-being.
Design: MASS Design Group in partnership with North Texas Family Health Foundation. Concept image courtesy of MASS Design Group

Empathy

Empathy, the ability to share in the experience of another creature and communicate that understanding, helps clinicians build stronger relationships with patients, improving patient satisfaction and clinical outcomes. The project-based learning approach of health design thinking can help medical students develop empathy, a known challenge in medical education.

When a health design team seeks to change the layout of a patient room or devise a new glucose monitor, they first try to understand the medical situation from diverse points of view. What's it like to be on the receiving end of a pelvic exam? Uncomfortable, embarrassing, and disempowering. The situation is even worse in emergency departments, where 6.3 million pelvic exams are performed annually—and gynecological beds are rarely available. Clinicians often improvise by pushing a bedpan under the person's pelvis. This workaround is demeaning to patients and can lead to suboptimal exams. When a team from the Health Design Lab began searching for a better way to perform pelvic exams in the ED, they knew they had to experience the exam process firsthand. The team included two male medical students, who put themselves on the exam table in order to understand the patient's perspective.

The design team also studied the problem of pelvic exams in the ED from the point of view of hospital administrators, who are concerned about cost and efficiency. It is expensive to transfer patients to stirrup-equipped beds elsewhere in the hospital. Existing wedge supports are bulky to store; even bulkier to store (and vastly more expensive) are full-sized, folding stirrup beds. In the process of making and testing prototypes and researching existing solutions, the team invented Tilt, a collapsible, portable wedge that is moderately priced, medically appropriate, and easy to store. Tilt also protects individual dignity and eases the workflow for caregivers.

Displaying your pelvis on a bedpan is one way to cultivate empathy. Designers also use interviews, observation, and role-playing to get closer to people's lives and learn from their expertise.

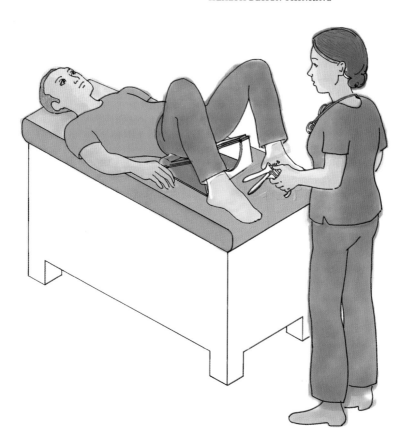

TILT is a portable medical device designed for performing pelvic exams in emergency departments. The team who designed the product includes three medical students, one occupational therapy student, and an industrial design student from Thomas Jefferson University. Understanding the experience of patients, doctors, and nurses was crucial to their design process. Historically, the medical field was dominated by men; today, more diverse perspectives are contributing to better products and protocols. The team founded the company Gia in order to develop their product for market. Design team: Sean Haynie, Hannah Levy, Elliott Perow, Kelly Sullivan, Sarah Weinblatt, Thomas Jefferson University

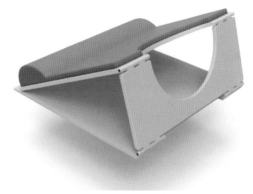

READ MORE Samantha A. Batt-Rawden, MBChB, *et al.*, "Teaching Empathy to Medical Students: An Updated, Systematic Review," *Academic Medicine* 88, no. 8 (2013): 1171–77, → doi: 10.1097/ACM.0b013e318299f3e3

BECOMING THE USER What challenges do individuals face in the realm of health care? Many new mothers must figure out how to pump breast milk frequently at work and in public places. Many older adults must learn how to take numerous medications with varying frequencies. People with diabetes may require multiple finger pricks daily. Like many aspects of the health care experience, these activities are neither intuitive nor easily described to others. When designers or clinicians try out a task themselves, their understanding becomes more concrete and embodied.

The process also can illuminate unmet needs and crystallize problems. Spend a few hours in a hospital waiting room. You might notice that you need a charging station for devices, or access to food for family members, or the ability to avoid close proximity with other patients while you are not feeling well.

The act of becoming the user allows designers and clinicians to identify challenges and experiences that may not be explicitly mentioned or even consciously known by the user. At Virginia Mason Medical Center in Seattle, a team of staff and clinicians was instructed by a consultant from Toyota in Japan to unfurl a spool of blue yarn over the map of the hospital along the path that a cancer patient would take. The blue yarn snaked across registration, laboratory, pharmacy, oncology, surgery, administrative, and financial offices. The knotty blue map that resulted showed how the current system demands excessive time and energy from some of the sickest patients. If the team had directly asked the patients to describe their experience of going to appointments, the patients might not have been able to convey the severity of the problem. Tracing the journey with blue yarn revealed the problem in a visceral way.

Onyx, a pharmaceutical company, asked SYPartners, a management consulting firm, to help them understand and enrich their own point of view toward patient-centered care. SYPartners told Onyx executives to locate and interview people with serious illnesses. Creative Director Thomas Winkelmann explains, "All SYPartners provided was a 'Be a Journalist for a Day' toolkit to guide them in going through their own contacts to get access to a patient and have a heartfelt, exploratory conversation. The executives had to find that person themselves. We weren't there when they met. It was a very humbling act for these business managers." The experience helped Onyx develop a deeper focus on patients—and to increase the company's funding of patient advocacy.

Many of the health care procedures one might seek to experience firsthand require access to the clinical care setting, which demands cooperation from medical teams. Plan how you will capture the insights learned from the exercise. Take care to document the experience and gather reflections that can be shared with others. Will someone film the interaction or record the sounds that are heard? Will you or someone else take photographs of key elements? When will you write down your raw reaction to the experience?

Your teammates may empathize with you more than they would with a stranger. Thus, when you share a video in which you are weary of tasting bitter medications or pricking your fingers multiple times a day, you become an advocate for your user, infecting your team with empathy.

The process has limitations, however. You will perceive and evaluate the activity based on your own values, biases, and experiences, as well as your own state of health. People most often experience health care when feeling unwell and unlike their normal selves—they may be anxious, scared, or harboring other feelings not fully present in your simulated experience. Seeking to understand a patient's viewpoint does not replace primary research, such as conducting interviews and surveys or co-creating with patients. Be mindful of your users' values and biases, and go through the experience knowing that you can never really wear another person's shoes.

READ MORE Charles Kenney, "The Blue Yarn," in *Transforming Health Care: Virginia Mason Medical Center's Pursuit of the Perfect Patient Experience* (CRC Press, 2011), 33–46.

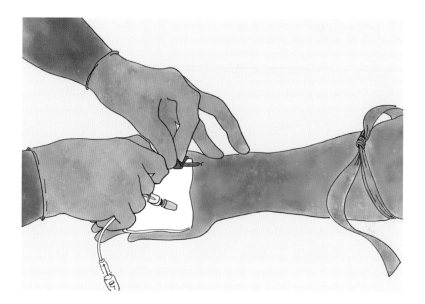

Find out how it feels to . . .

Find your way through a hospital complex without asking for directions.

Sleep in the emergency department to simulate the experience of a patient waiting for a hospital bed after being admitted.

Stay overnight in an inpatient bed and get your vital signs checked every four hours.

Concentrate on a difficult task in the doctor's workspace in a busy outpatient clinic.

Get an intravenous line started on you (above).

Navigate the hospital with a wheelchair, walker, or cane, or with crutches.

Arrive in an ambulance as a "trauma activation," wherein the trauma team descends upon you to perform an initial trauma resuscitation.

Wear a hospital gown.

Test your blood sugar three times a day.

Remember to bring an item such as an EpiPen with you—everywhere.

Take a complex set of placebos—some twice a day and some three times a day.

Taste the medications commonly prescribed to children. They are surprisingly bitter!

Codesign

Empathy is a crucial component of human-centered design. But empathy alone is not enough. Focusing exclusively on empathy can lead to separating "us" (designers and health care professionals) from "them" (users and patients). Patients and other stakeholders should be active participants in the design process, not just objects of empathic feeling. Individuals who experience ailments, injuries, or disabilities are experts on their own life condition. Codesign is a collaborative process that actively seeks knowledge and ideas from end users.

Each member of a design team has deep knowledge about their own life experience. Codesign directly injects this expertise into the design process. Furthermore, team members have diverse and overlapping areas of knowledge. A patient may also be a design professional, a clinician, a health expert, or an advocate.

Codesign should be integral to the design, execution, and interpretation of research. Currently, patient involvement is not yet routine in biomedical and health services research. Dr. Kristin Rising, a researcher and physician at Thomas Jefferson University, embeds patients as active and equal participants on her research teams. In one study that she led, patients on the research team enrolled study participants, conducted interviews, led group brainstorming sessions, and performed data analysis. The team developed a list of patient goals related to seeking care for diabetes. Having real patients on the study team enabled all researchers to understand their subject from a patient perspective. Patient voices were present during the gathering, analysis, and final interpretation of data. Involving patients and the public is required for funding many research studies and clinical trials.

Tools for codesign include user interviews, photo journals, surveys, and user testing in addition to inclusive brainstorming activities. Each co-creation process should be executed in a way that acknowledges the expertise of all participants. Codesign takes effort. Patients must be willing and able to contribute their time and expertise. Care must be taken to avoid reverting to familiar power structures or exploiting the experiences of people who are vulnerable or have survived trauma.

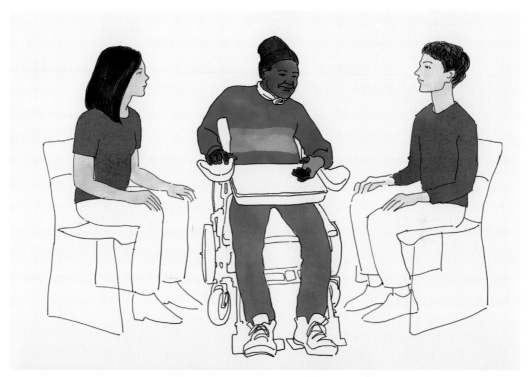

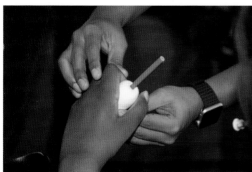

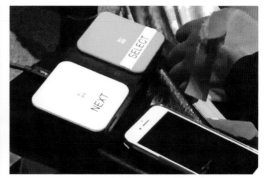

TEAM WORK Students in design, medicine, and pharmacy at Thomas Jefferson University codesigned tools with Lariq Byrd to create custom tools. Byrd breathes with a ventilator and uses a wheel chair for mobility. Maximizing subtle movements in his left hand and wrist is important to his quality of life. Byrd participated in each step of the design process, including defining the problem, teaching the team about the issue, and testing and retesting prototypes. Together, the team created products uniquely suited to Byrd's abilities, including a remote control that responds to micro movements and a glove designed to optimize Byrd's grip.

READ MORE Elizabeth B.-N. Sanders and Pieter Jan Stappers, *Convivial Toolbox: Generative Research for the Front End of Design* (Amsterdam: BIS Publishers, 2012); Deana McDonagh, "Design Students Forseeing the Unforeseeable: Practice-Based Empathic Research Methods," *International Journal of Education through Art* 11, no. 3 (2015), doi:10.1386/eta.11.3.421_1; Dr. Kristin Rising, → www.pcori.org/research-results/2015/concept-mapping-scalable-method-identifying-patient-important-outcomes

DESIGN FOR ONE Codesign allows for the generation of customized solutions for individuals who have unique challenges. Open Style Lab (OSL), led by Grace Jun, uses codesign to help people living with disabilities perform to their full capacities. OSL raises awareness of accessible style through public events and workshops.

Clothing is an essential tool used by humans to engage and integrate with their environments and communities. Lack of access to adaptive clothing diminishes the dignity and independence of people with disabilities.

An OSL team member, Kieran Kern is a freelance writer, advocate, and mom who has cerebral palsy. Kieran desired stylish clothing that she could wear to client meetings and could put on and remove without the assistance of others. The design team created an attractive, functional red coat with a silk lining, batwing sleeves, a rigid collar insert, and armholes with a large circumference. The design allows Kern to easily bring the coat around the back of her shoulders and insert her arms into the sleeves. The garment is professional but not too formal. It provides warmth, and—perhaps most important—it embodies Kern's spirit and positive energy.

OSL addresses the gap in the current market for adaptive clothing and wearable technologies. In the U.S., one out of five people identify as having a disability, but few companies offer products that adequately address accessibility. This population is often lumped into one group without consideration for the unique conditions and needs of individuals. To reduce inequality and foster inclusive design innovation, OSL offers programs where codesign flourishes. Designers, engineers, and occupational therapists work with a person with a disability to make functional clothing and accessories that are also fashionable.

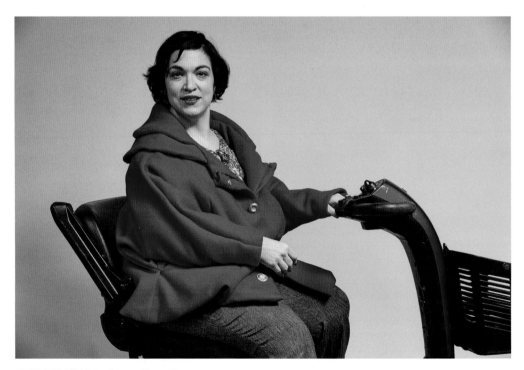

OPEN STYLE LAB Designers: Kieran Kern, Magdalena Kraszpulska, Noah Litvin, Xiaojie Yang, and Tong Zhang.

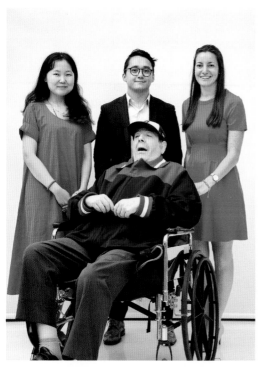

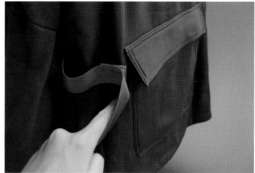

ON AND OFF Softable is a jacket designed to be donned and doffed independently by a user with limited upper body strength and range of motion. The OSL team developed a unique garment fitted with 3D-printed snaps and a pulley for cinching the waist. Instead of using zippers or buttons, Robert prefers to pull the garment over his head, but that can leave the garment too loose in the stomach area. Thus, the team designed a waist belt built into the garment. Robert is able to pull the belt with his dexterity, reach, and strength. Designers: Alyssa Brandofino, Bolor Amgalan, Herbert Ramirez, and Robert Appelman, the Riverside Premier Rehabilitation and Healing Center in New York City

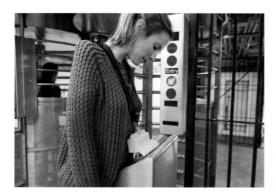

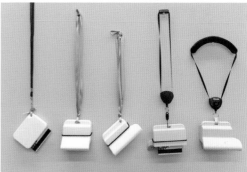

HANDS FREE Patients living with amyotrophic lateral sclerosis (ALS), or Lou Gehrig's disease, face daily challenges in their routine lives—brushing their hair, typing on a computer, or eating meals. Christina Mallon, a woman working as an inclusive experience designer at Wunderman Thompson, has a rare form of ALS that has left her arms and hands completely paralyzed. The progressive loss of function of her hands and arms over the years has made daily activities like dressing and taking transportation extremely difficult. The OSL design team created Swipe, a 3D-printed portable device that allows Christina to push her Metrocard through the card reader at a subway turnstile. Swipe hangs around the neck and attaches to the turnstile by tiny magnets. Without Swipe, Christina could not ride the subway independently and would risk losing her job because of not being able to commute to work. This solution is customized to her unique needs and lifestyle. Designers: OSL team (Christina Mallon, Julia Liao), Estee Bruno, Claudia Poh, and Ultimaker.

Social Determinants

Modern societies place a tremendous burden on individuals to safeguard their health. The behaviors connected with a "healthy lifestyle" are held up as matters of personal virtue, yet people are constantly confronted with cheap, addictive food options and sedentary activities. Rich people live in areas with clean air, clean water, and open green spaces, while people experiencing poverty occupy dangerous neighborhoods that are devoid of opportunity.

Health, like wealth, is distributed unevenly. Social determinants of health include food, housing, education, employment, and transportation as well as medical care. Low-income communities, like groups facing discrimination based on race, gender, sexuality, or disability, often lack access to health-enhancing resources. The persistent bias experienced by marginalized groups further degrades health and leads to lower-quality care within health care systems that perpetuate bias.

Recognizing social determinants is a crucial aspect of health care. Expanding on the particularity of each person's unique experience, health design thinking considers the broader demographic factors that cause health inequality. Looking beyond the individual, we begin to understand health care in terms of social, cultural, and economic systems. Health design thinking is a tool that hospital administrators can use to address the social determinants of health, which have tremendous economic consequences.

Many social determinants of health are connected to the design of our physical environments. In countless cities around the world, design decisions favor cars and elevators over sidewalks and stairways. Inadequate public transit and segregated housing trap people in poverty. Multilane roadways cut through underinvested communities, causing pedestrian injuries and fatalites from cars. Rural areas lack hospitals and clinics. Cigarettes and processed foods contribute to global problems of obesity, diabetes, and lung and heart disease. Design thinking can be a tool for seeking health across communities and diminishing health inequities.

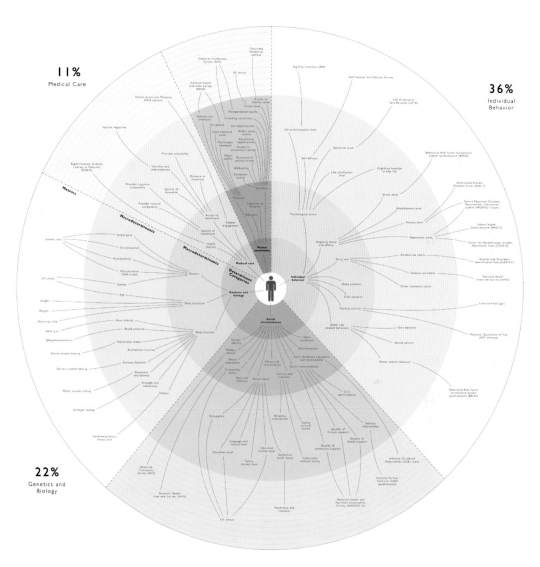

HEALTH FACTORS (full-size detail on following pages) Working with research and statistics gathered from numerous scientific sources and public agencies, the design firm GoInvo mapped out factors correlated with an individual's health outcomes. The behaviors of an individual are often guided and constrained by social conditions. Design: GoInvo

READ MORE Laura K. Brennan Ramirez, PhD, MPH, Elizabeth A. Baker, PhD, MPH, and Marilyn Metzler, RN, *Promoting Health Equity: A Resource to Help Communities Address Social Determinants of Health* (Centers for Disease Control and Prevention, 2008).

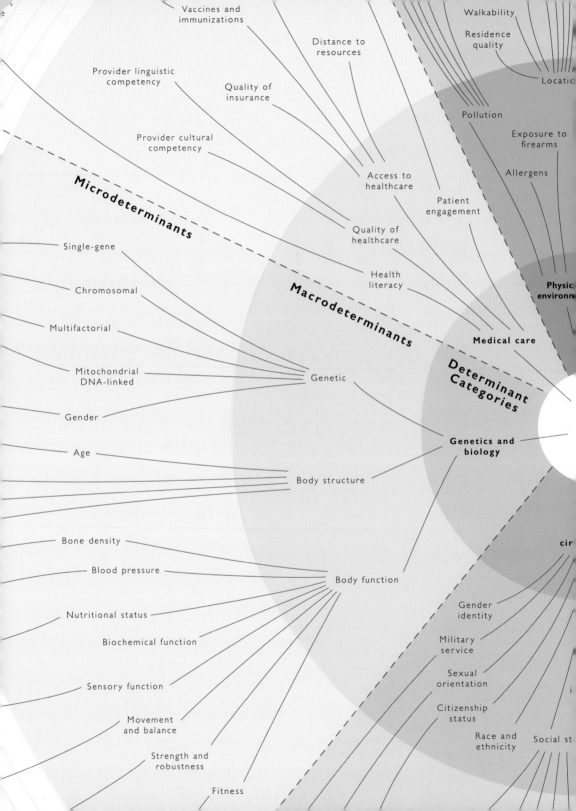

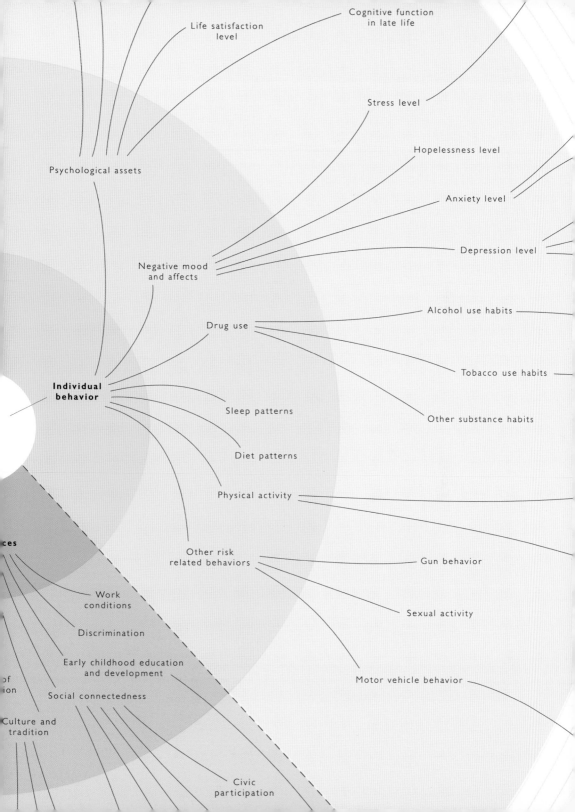

Cognitive function
in late life

Life satisfaction
level

Stress level

Hopelessness level

Psychological assets

Anxiety level

Depression level

Negative mood
and affects

Alcohol use habits

Drug use

Tobacco use habits

Individual
behavior

Other substance habits

Sleep patterns

Diet patterns

Physical activity

Gun behavior

Other risk
related behaviors

Sexual activity

ces

Work
conditions

Discrimination

Early childhood education
and development

of
ion

Social connectedness

Motor vehicle behavior

Culture and
tradition

Civic
participation

CONNECTING COMMUNITIES WITH RESOURCES

In many communities, there is a profound gap between available health care resources and the people who could benefit from them. Services may exist that are used to full capacity. An older adult needing home care may not know how to register for visiting nursing services. The parent of a child with asthma may be overwhelmed by the task of eliminating asthma triggers from the family's home. A young adult derailed by depression, anxiety, or substance abuse may struggle to find treatment. A person experiencing unstable housing may lack access to medications for a chronic condition. An undocumented immigrant may avoid applying for health care services.

Various organizations have used design thinking to help bridge the gap between health care resources and individuals in need. Processes that combine digital tools with active, person-to-person outreach can help people address obstacles to better health.

NowPow, a tool and community network created in Chicago, aims to connect people with care resources in their communities. Dr. Stacy Lindau, cofounder of NowPow, developed the concept of creating an electronic prescription for community-based resources. She calls this principle "e-prescribing community" or CommunityRx. At the core of NowPow is a health information technology platform that is integrated with electronic record systems used in over thirty clinical sites in Chicago. This digital platform allows clinicians, social workers, and other care clinicians to match individuals with resources in their neighborhoods.

Health design interventions fail when they are imposed from the top down, without regard for a community's own expertise, priorities, values, and resources. Sending patients to a website or handing them a brochure is useless in the absence of a full process of engagement that yields mutual respect and understanding.

A health intervention must be viable in its local context. In the U.S., many rural communities lack easy access to the internet. In many developing regions around the world, cell phones are widely used for banking and business, whereas desktop computers are rare. In other regions, Facebook is the primary means of interacting online. Literacy, education, and attitudes toward sexuality and reproduction are other important factors in designing successful tools for health care.

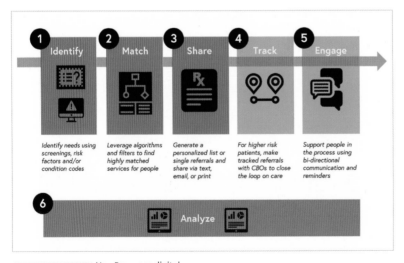

COMMUNITY HEALTH NowPow uses digital and human resources to connect clinicians with people in need of services.

BUILDING UNDERSTANDING Misinformation or distrust can lead individuals and communities to underutilize an available health resource. The Baltimore City Health Department (BCHD) sought to increase access to long-acting reversible contraceptives (LARCs). The goal was to achieve "contraceptive equity"—meaning that all people should be able to choose, obtain, and use any FDA-approved contraceptive for family planning and the prevention of sexually transmitted infections.

Over a several-year period, the LARC Access Project expanded availability of LARCs in publicly funded family planning clinics, trained over 500 clinical staff and providers, and contributed to the increase in LARC utilization from 10% to 20% throughout Baltimore City. Despite these advances, the BCHD needed to address client demand. Creating better access to a health care resource isn't useful if people don't know about it or don't want to use it. As clinics improve LARC access, they must also address the prevalence of provider mistrust, birth control myths, and lack of health education.

In 2018, the Center for Social Design at MICA (Maryland Institute College of Art) began working with BCHD to understand the barriers to family planning in Baltimore and develop prototypes for educational materials. The design process was informed by surveys and interviews collected from various stakeholders, including Baltimore City women, family planning medical providers, and leaders and staff from a community outreach organization (B'more for Healthy Babies).

The design team prototyped a Family Planning Toolkit for use in counseling sessions. Designed to support lively, hands-on discussions, the Toolkit aims to guide women's perceptions of contraceptives and encourage them to choose more effective birth control methods. Bright, playful, and accessible, the Toolkit uses gamelike activities and informative graphics to prompt reflection on family planning decision-making and address common barriers, such as myths and misconceptions, challenges with access to services, provider mistrust, and male partner engagement. The Toolkit also addresses overall goal setting and pregnancy planning.

Projects like this view health care as more than a technical service. Effective medical interventions must meet the needs of a community and be created through an active and respectful process of listening and learning.

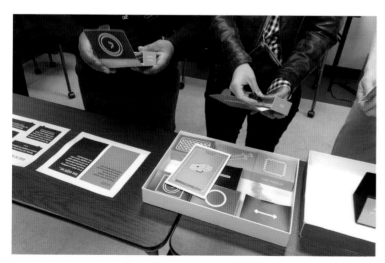

FAMILY PLANNING TOOLKIT Project leads, MICA's Center for Social Design: Charlotte Hager and Becky Slogeris. Project team, MICA's Center for Social Design: Hayelin Choi, Sarah Dunn, Elishabha Eaton, Aylin Onur, Vic Liu, Claudia Norena, Rachel Serra, Amber Summers, Jade Shih, Cecilia Yang. Advisors: Denise Shanté Brown, Alexandra Eisler, Vanessa Geffrard, Dr. Olnfunke Pickering, and Dr. Nishant Shah. Partner: Baltimore City Department of Health.

Creative Mindset

Creativity is not a rare talent. It is a fundamental human capacity that anyone can cultivate. Specific techniques and exercises can wake up the thought processes and help us generate ideas more easily. Most ideas disappear unless we write them down or make a sketch. An idea that lives only inside our own heads rarely lasts long or travels far. As we love and care for an idea—adding details and exploring its consequences—a fleeting thought becomes a concrete concept that can be discussed, tested, or even built. A few basic principles guide the process of generating ideas and making them concrete:

QUESTIONING is the act of looking at any problem from a new angle. It is the process of asking questions and reframing assumptions. A good question helps us look at a situation and ask, "How could this be different?"

VISUALIZING draws on our innate ability to perceive objects and spaces, patterns and structures. Designers use line, shape, color, and form to make connections, reveal insights, and communicate concepts.

PROTOTYPING is the act of making ideas concrete in a provisional, speculative way. Although some prototypes resemble real products or include a working mechanism, many prototypes are rough sketches or quickly assembled artifacts that explore one aspect of a proposed design solution.

STORYTELLING is the universal art of recounting a signficant action that takes place over time. Designers gather stories from users and other stakeholders, and they create stories about how a product, space, or service will be used and experienced.

A well-prepared mind is equipped to unleash creativity and come up with new ideas. When (according to legend) Archimedes shouted "Eureka" in his bathtub, he was able to do so because he had been thinking long and hard about the problem of how to measure volume. In the process of health design thinking, a period of careful, attentive research prepares our minds for active making and discovery.

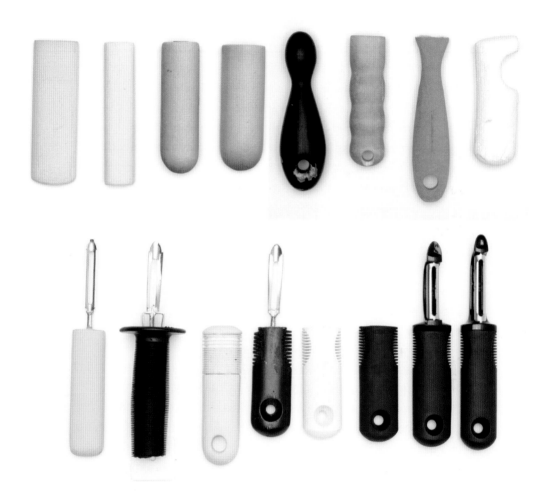

PROTOTYPES FOR OXO GOOD GRIPS PEELER

The OXO brand was born when Betsey and Sam Farber set out to create better kitchen tools for people who experience pain when gripping hard, narrow handles. Betsey was an architect and Sam was a kitchenware designer. Betsey had arthritis, which made it difficult for her to use many standard tools. The Farbers partnered with Smart Design, who created dozens of handle prototypes out of wood, rubber, plastic, and foam. They also borrowed handles from existing products, including a black rubber bicycle handle. When the design team laid out their prototypes on a table, people kept picking up the bicycle handle, delighting in its warm, sturdy feel. Today, the OXO Good Grips brand encompasses numerous products, including medical devices. The black rubber handle has become an icon of comfort and ease of use. Design: Smart Design with Betsey and Sam Farber. Manufactured by OXO (USA). Stainless steel, Santoprene (thermoplastic rubber), carved foam, plastic, wood, plaster, polypropylene, graphite on preprinted white wove paper. Collection of Cooper Hewitt, Smithsonian Design Museum, 1992-52-1/10, 25; 2011-50-1/9, 11/20; 2011-50-24. READ MORE about Betsey Farber in a 2018 essay by Liz Jackson, "We Are the Original Lifehackers," at www.nytimes.com/2018/05/30/opinion/disability-design-lifehacks.html.

Questioning

Questioning is the act of viewing any problem from a new angle. This process helps us reframe assumptions. Looking at problems from different perspectives is a crucial tool in the process of both design and medicine. The questions in health care are complex. The answers are rarely black-and-white, yet physicians are trained to make a definitive diagnosis and treat the illness. However, problems in health care systems—ranging from how to expand access to primary care to how to reduce medical errors—are difficult to fix using medicine's traditional mindsets. Although the evidence-based approach to disease has been successful in biomedical research, it fails to address many of the challenges in health care. The hypothesis-driven scientific method assumes that you know exactly which questions to ask. But more often than not, we ask the wrong questions. Design thinking starts with identifying the problem in an open-ended way that doesn't predetermine the answer.

Health design thinking can provide a framework for tackling chronic diseases such as diabetes. A patient who struggles with controlling her blood sugar requires more than a doctor's instructions on the optimal insulin regimen and low-carbohydrate diet. Asking "Why?" expands understanding and invites people to share their stories. Their answers will show that the social determinants of health play a huge role in managing diabetes and other chronic medical conditions. A patient may reveal that she can no longer afford insulin because of a new insurance plan or that feelings of social isolation leave her less motivated to monitor her glucose levels.

Instead of labeling patients as noncompliant when they don't carry out our prescribed treatment plans, clinicians can work with patients to design treatments that have a higher probability of succeeding. For example, if a person with diabetes presents with elevated blood glucose levels arising from unhealthy eating behaviors, asking open-ended questions can illuminate the challenge from a patient's point of view: "What kind of problems are you having with your diet?" "What's the worst part of eating unhealthy?" "What do you hope for?"

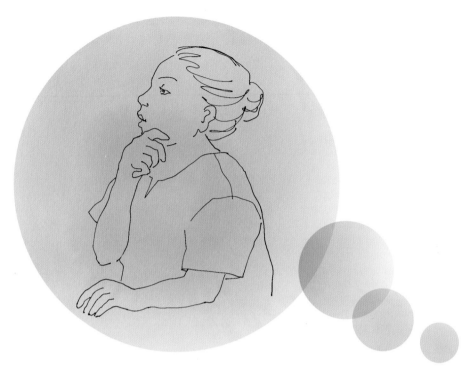

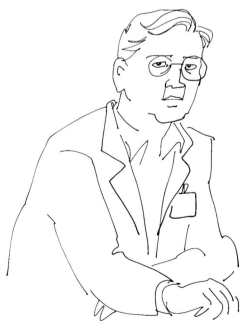

Asking and listening

Deeper insight into the human condition can transform patient narratives.

Medical documentation in the electronic health record (EHR) describes patients like this: *Susan is a 33-year-old insulin-dependent diabetic female who has noncompliant behavior, including difficulty adhering to dietary recommendations.*

Looking at a person from a new angle can humanize the patient: *Susan, a busy, single, working mother of two toddlers living with type 2 diabetes, eats fast food every night because she's too exhausted to cook a meal and lacks access to local healthy food options. Medications are too expensive for her budget.*

HOW-MIGHT-WE QUESTIONS The design thinking methodology developed by IDEO and the Stanford d.school features a special way to frame a design problem. Called a "how-might-we question," or HMW, this query helps open the mind for creative thinking. An HMW is narrow enough to prompt people to develop specific, focused ideas; at the same time, it is broad enough that it doesn't limit concepts around a predetermined outcome.

The HMWs shown on the opposite page were created in a workshop led by the Health Design Lab at Thomas Jefferson University with employees at IMRE, a marketing agency with a focus on health care. Workshop participants were asked to imagine new products or services for patients who had just received a diagnosis of diabetes. Role-playing exercises helped participants imagine receiving this diagnosis themselves. Participants also discussed the illness with one of the workshop leaders—a clinical pharmacist who himself has diabetes. They also experienced the challenge of using a blood glucose monitor for the first time.

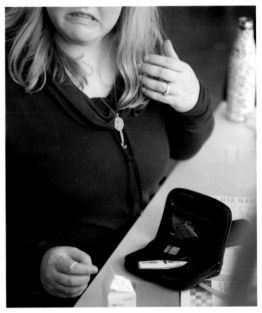

Photo: David Campbell

How might we?

Fruitful questions for a design challenge focus on a specific aspect of a user's experience. Look for questions that are open-ended rather than ones that suggest a particular solution in advance.

> **How might we...**
> TRANSFORM THE MOMENT of DIAGNOSIS
>
> **so that....**
> the patient feels empowered to tackle their new normal.

FOCUS: EXPERIENCING THE INITIAL DIAGNOSIS

Big questions for the future of health care

The questions listed below were generated by the Kyu Collective, a group of diverse creative companies committed to addressing the most significant challenges facing business and society. These visionary questions were framed during a workshop addressing the future of wellness. The questions do not presume a particular type of solution, which leaves us free to imagine future practices very different from those of today. Each question suggests many other questions, opening up rich areas for creative thinking.

How might we connect our personal health to the health of the planet?

How might we strive for a culture of vitality?

How might we think of health as a social contract?

How might we create new currencies that can be used as incentives?

How does human and tech add up to more than the sum?

Who owns you?

Is the goal of health immortality?

How might we create fulfilling, sustainable, restorative roles for providers (and beyond)?

How might we create health communities (online and offline) that are joyful, inclusive, and seamless, that people truly want?

How might we engage a team of diverse health care "supporters" around the delivery of lifelong, holistic care?

How might we enable a scalable symphony of high-touch and high-tech care across the journey of lifelong health?

What happens when bioelectronics and bionic augmentation replace drugs?

Visualizing

Visualizing ideas and information is a bedrock of design practice. The process of creating a drawing, diagram, or physical model can lead to discoveries and insights. Sketching is a powerful way to find relationships and generate ideas. Clear, direct graphics help people explain and illuminate concepts. Shapes, colors, illustrations, and typography are the basic ingredients of welcoming, purposeful communications.

For humans and other creatures, vision is an active process for making sense of the environment. From a flood of perceptual data, we recognize distinct objects and events. We seek out patterns and register change. The human eye darts about the field of vision, building moving pictures of the world. Sometimes, we use vision to complete a task—such as reading a line of text or finding an anomaly on an X-ray. In other instances, we explore the environment more freely. While walking through a city, we glance around at people and buildings and experience the peripheral movement of traffic.

Designers rely on visual thinking, and so do doctors and nurses. Symptoms can reveal themselves through bodily signs that are visible—and tactual—to the experienced eye and hand. Medical illustrations help clinicians understand the inner workings of the body. X-rays, sonograms, and CT scans allow care teams to peer beneath the surface. In office visits, clinicians use drawings, photographs, and models to explain procedures to patients. More recently, 3D-printed models of hearts and other organs—customized for individuals— have become tools for planning surgery.

Visual thinking isn't just for individuals with excellent eyesight. Many people who experience blindness or low vision are avid visual thinkers, who prefer tactile graphics and 3D models over lengthy linear descriptions. Data visualization is a powerful application of visual thinking. Many people have trouble evaluating statistics when they are presented in a strictly numerical fashion.

Using color to express information

CONVENTIONAL COLOR

Social conventions allow colors to have certain meanings in certain situations. The colors of traffic signals and road signs are used consistently in most parts of the world. Such conventions also function in medical contexts.

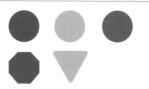

CONVENTIONAL COLORS FOR TRAFFIC SIGNS

ARBITRARY COLOR

When sorting ideas or creating a data graphic, designers create systems that assign colors to different variables or categories of information. Office dot stickers are useful for prototyping products and for labeling files.

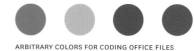

ARBITRARY COLORS FOR CODING OFFICE FILES

COLOR TO CONVEY DATA

Colors can represent numbers or values when they are arranged in a sequence from warm to cool, dark to light, or brilliant to pastel. A monochrome color system uses one hue, such as blue, in different shades. A polychrome system uses two or more colors, such as blue and orange to represent temperature.

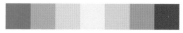

COLOR SYSTEM REPRESENTING TEMPERATURE

COLOR AND FEELING This design for a digital app allows patients to track their pain levels. The design relies on illustrations and color instead of written language. Colors ranging from bright yellow to dark red express the concept of pain intensity in a manner that is more intuitive to understand than a traditional numerical pain scale. Design: GoInvo

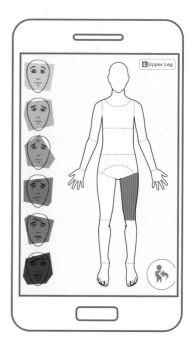

SPATIAL DATA Data visualizations do more than make information easier to understand. They reveal patterns and connections that might otherwise go unnoticed. Understanding the basic principles of visual design can help any design thinker communicate in ways that are easy for others to grasp—and bring new insights to light.

Designers at GoInvo sketched the diagram below to map an individual's personality as measured by the Myers-Briggs Type Indicator (MBTI), an instrument that is widely used for assessing personality preferences. Typically, MBTI results are represented with a set of initials, such as ENFJ, for *extravert*, *intuitive*, *feeling*, and

judging. These compact initials fail to show us personality preferences in relation to each other. The pen-and-pencil sketch created by GoInvo maps numbers onto a radial grid, thereby showing how an individual responded to diverse questions.

Dense pages of data are a fact of life in the medical professions. The health history of a patient can consist of many pages of documents. For clinicians, making sense of these documents demands time and endurance. For patients, explaining their health histories to multiple clinicians can be deeply frustrating. Katie McCurdy, founder of Pictal Health, collaborates with patients to create visual timelines of their

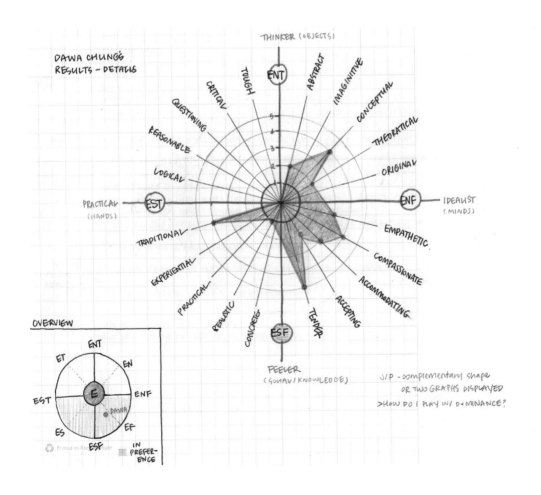

health. Timelines like the one shown below enable patients and clinicians to perceive relationships between symptoms, treatments, and life events, and to see small bits of data as parts of a larger whole. McCurdy's graphics are both functional and illuminating. A reader can search for specific information, such as "When did we diagnose GERD?" A reader can also look at the whole pattern or Gestalt of the timeline and see that symptoms spike around life events.

McCurdy's graphics make skillful use of visual design elements, such as color, size, transparency, and typography. Each main category has its own color group: purple for symptoms,

yellow for life events, and blue for diagnoses and treatments. Colors overlap and mix with each other (transparency) to indicate simultaneous events.

Text labels are placed next to the data they identify, reducing the need for a separate key. Bold headings invite quick scanning. A single size of type is used throughout the body of the timeline, eliminating unnecessary complexity. A timeline like this one can help the health care team avoid repeating ineffective treatments and tests.

Learn more about information design: Method | Data Visualization. Learn more about Pictal Health: Case Study | Visual Health History.

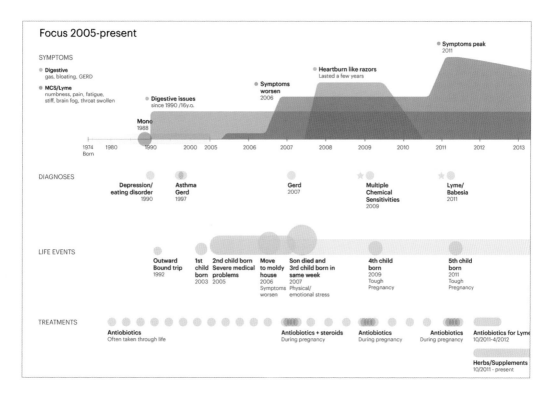

PERSONALITY MAP (opposite) This radial diagram represents the results of a Myers-Briggs Type Indicator test in a comprehensive visual manner. Design: GoInvo

HEALTH HISTORY TIMELINE (detail) A patient's experience comes into focus with the aid of a visual graph. Doctor and patient alike can make better sense of a complex history when its elements are laid out in a clear visual format. Design: Katie McCurdy, Pictal Health

DRAWING AND SKETCHING Drawing is a form of thinking. Just as talking with a colleague or taking notes helps us articulate an idea and give it shape, drawing is a process of discovery and making. Not every drawing needs to be perfect. Quick sketches communicate the feeling of a work in progress. Complex works of architecture often begin with gestural sketches indicating a central idea. Sketches of people using a device offer points of departure for discussion and further development.

Biomedical illustrations are used in the context of medical textbooks, pharmaceutical marketing, medical device development, medical forensics, patient education, and more. Employing traditional drawing and painting techniques as well as 3D rendering and animation, biomedical illustrations often represent structures the human eye cannot detect. Amanda S. Almon, professor of biomedical art and visualization at Rowan University, calls her field "Pixar for medicine."

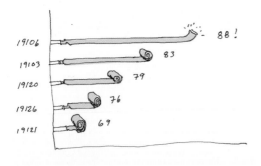

ZIP CODE GAP Chris Landau created this graph to illustrate the disparity of life expectancies among people living in different zip codes in Philadelphia, Pennsylvania. Access to a healthy environment helps people in richer communities live a longer life.

INSIDIOUS INFECTION This stunning visualization by Amanda S. Almon, CMI (Certified Medical Illustrator), depicts the unseen process of a cellular infection. Bacteria invade the protective phospholipid bilayer while innate immune (B-cells) line up for a defensive barrier. This image is a still frame from an educational animation about genetic immunity.

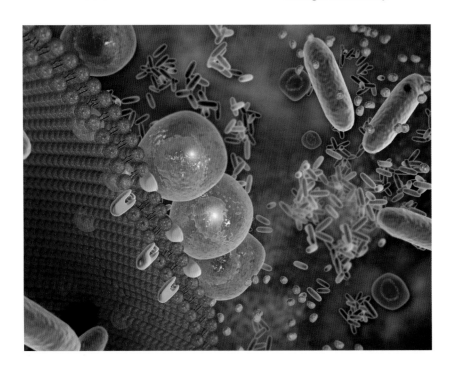

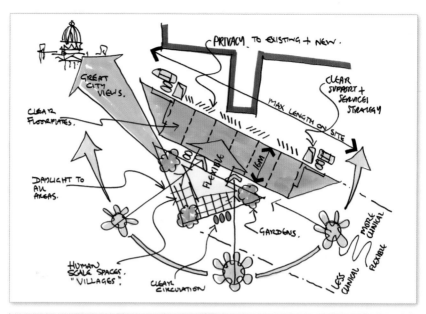

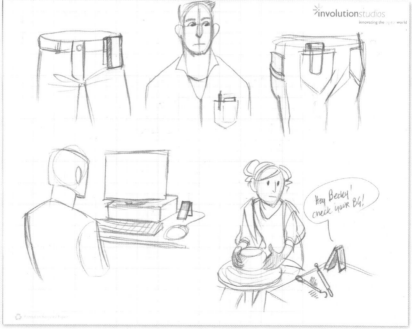

CANCER CENTRE AT GUY'S HOSPITAL (top) In this sketch for a London cancer center, the Treatment Zone is gray, and the more public, social Care Zone is yellow. Drawing: Ivan Harbour/Rogers Stirk Harbour + Partners

SKETCHING SCENARIOS (bottom) These drawings show how users might employ a device in their daily lives. The informal style keeps us focused on the general idea rather than on specific product styling. Design: GoInvo

Prototyping

Prototyping gives physical shape and form to our ideas. Insights gained through observing users and imagining solutions take form as tangible products or processes. Prototypes help us not only to communicate our ideas but also to allow others to experience them and give feedback. Although many people see prototyping as an activity reserved for engineers who build complex machines like vehicles or computers, prototyping is a surprisingly simple and universal activity. Anyone can do it! Prototypes do not have to be high tech. Sketches, storyboards, physical mock-ups, role-playing, and simulation are methods for fleshing out ideas and finding out how a potential design solution could affect people.

Prototyping is fundamental to developing new medical devices and to improving health care services and creating better patient experiences. Sharing rough ideas and early concepts might feel uncomfortable at first. Clinicians are not accustomed to showing their work to others in its early stages; they often spend weeks and even months developing new hospital protocols and workflows before soliciting feedback. As a process, prototyping can make us more comfortable with failing and prevent us from getting attached to a single solution. Exploring the improvisational spirit of prototyping is an invaluable experience for any medical professional.

Prototyping fuels the creative process through making—it enables us to think with our hands. Prototyping is iterative, allowing us not just to model objects, services, and settings but also to learn and improve upon the interactions among all these conditions.

Materials for each prototyping form vary in cost and complexity. Inexpensive prototypes are particularly useful in early stages, where the flexibility to scrap, repurpose, and remodel quickly can allow for creativity in design and new directions. For example, if you have an idea for a new mobile app that supports mental health in patients, try prototyping it yourself through sketching. You don't need to be a software engineer or know how to write a single line of code in order to develop an app prototype—you just need pen and paper.

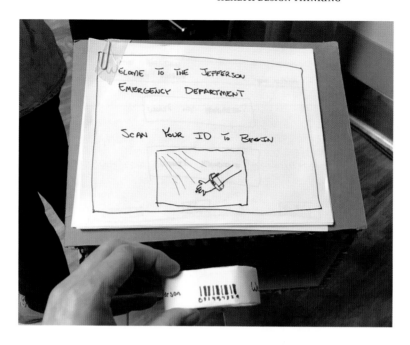

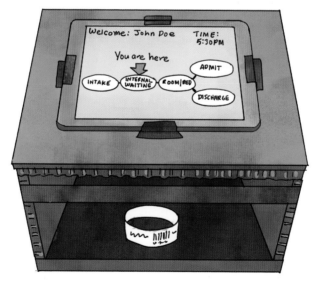

PROTOTYPE FOR A DIGITAL APP These prototypes represent a kiosk that gives patients real-time updates on their status in the ED. By scanning the barcode on their ID wristbands, patients can view results of their labs and understand what diagnostic imaging is pending. The first prototype (top) uses paper sketches of screen flows to plan out the interaction. In the second prototype (bottom), a digital sketch has been loaded onto a tablet.

PROTOTYPING WITH OBJECTS In a design workshop for the medical packaging industry, the Health Design Lab at Thomas Jefferson University challenged interdisciplinary teams composed of engineers, corporate managers and suppliers, physicians, nurses, and technicians to create a better central line experience. Central lines or central venous catheters are large tubes that are inserted in vessels going to the heart; they deliver fluids and medications to critically ill or unstable patients. Infections associated with central lines are a leading cause of death in hospitals.

After workshop participants interviewed each other and were shown how to insert a central line, teams were prompted to create a better central line experience in two ways: through role-playing and through physical prototyping. Role-playing allows you to experience a prototype or existing product. Participants quickly uncovered critical shortcomings of the standard central line kit by physically simulating the procedure. Current packaging with small print makes it difficult to know the contents of the procedure kit and whether any supplemental items are required. To make it easier for a physician to safely complete the procedure, a team role-played a potential solution where the essential items for central line insertion were color-coded with stickers for easier identification.

Building physical prototypes for a redesigned central line experience inspired a wide range of creative ideas. In addressing the problem of disorganization within central line kits, one team used a combination of Legos, duct tape, and plastic toys to design a foldout package that separated major steps—sterile prep, catheter placement, and sharps disposal—into geographically distinct areas with clear labels. Another team created a hanging organizer that arranges equipment sequentially in a long strip to minimize the need to search through a tray of sharp materials; this prototype makes it easier to visualize and identify what is needed when doing the procedure. Other prototypes include a central line kit with outer compartments containing essential items (sterile gloves, caps for catheter ports, and a mini sharps container) and a deconstructed kit that that could be customized for a specific clinical department. Prototyping helped teams imagine solutions that could make the procedure safer and more efficient, reducing the incidence of needlestick injuries.

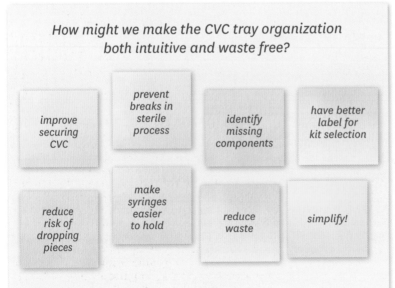

How might we make the CVC tray organization both intuitive and waste free?

improve securing CVC

prevent breaks in sterile process

identify missing components

have better label for kit selection

reduce risk of dropping pieces

make syringes easier to hold

reduce waste

simplify!

HOW MIGHT WE? Questions like these are generated in brainstorming sessions and informed by user interviews and observations. These questions guide the prototyping process.

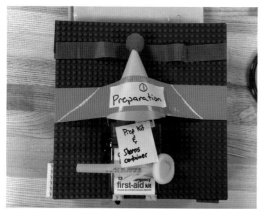

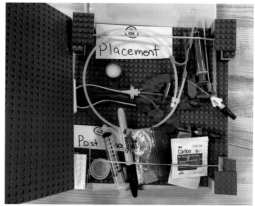

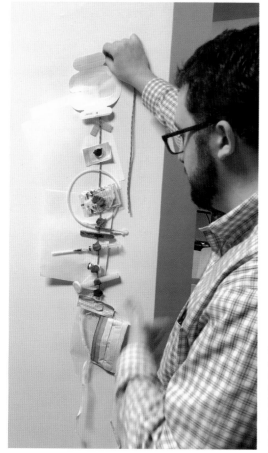

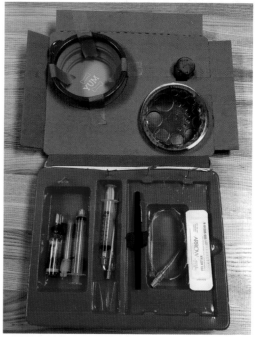

CENTRAL LINE KIT PROTOTYPES (top left) A surgical cap and extra items for skin preparation are attached to the outside of the kit. (top right) When the doctor opens the kit, the contents are organized sequentially. (bottom left) In this deconstructed, customized central line kit, the critical components needed for the procedure are laid out, helping to prevent the routine disposal of unnecessary items. (bottom right) This design arranges items in intuitive, geographic compartments. A dog water bowl represents a sharps disposal container that can be embedded into the lid of the foldout kit.

PROTOTYPING WITH PAPER A team of medical students and emergency medicine physicians tackled the challenge of improving sepsis care at Thomas Jefferson University Hospital. They discovered a common thread among sepsis cases that could have gone better: failed communication. Problems ranged from communication breakdowns between doctors and nurses to alarm fatigue, message fatigue in the EHR, and poor transitions of care between the ED and inpatient hospital teams.

The design team prototyped a visual checklist to help the emergency care team perform the critical actions in sepsis management. Doing this allowed them to gain immediate feedback from nurses, technicians, and physicians in the ED. Instead of spending months trying to figure out how to develop a solution that could be embedded in the existing computer system, they were able to gain valuable insight from a paper prototype.

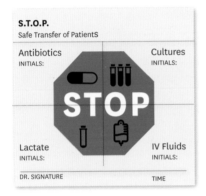

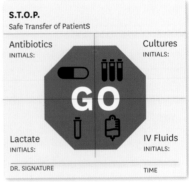

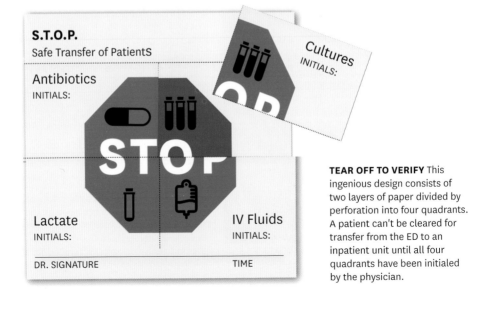

TEAR OFF TO VERIFY This ingenious design consists of two layers of paper divided by perforation into four quadrants. A patient can't be cleared for transfer from the ED to an inpatient unit until all four quadrants have been initialed by the physician.

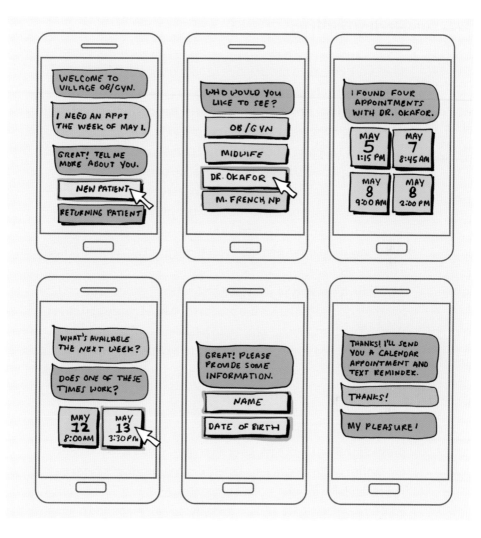

PAPER MOCK-UPS Digital apps can be prototyped with sketches on paper. Templates for sketching a sequence of digital screens are easily found online. The sketch above describes a potential interaction with a chatbot interface designed for scheduling a medical appointment via text message. Paper sketches like this one become the basis for more refined digital prototypes that can be tested and discussed with users.

Storytelling

Stories are crucial to the practice of both design and medicine. A story consists of a significant action taking place over time. A story has a beginning, a middle, and an end. It has characters and settings that engage our senses and stir our emotions. A story's action leads to change in circumstances (solving a crime, completing a quest, confronting a past trauma, or finding a life partner, for example).

Designers use color, texture, and imagery to set the mood of a brand, a publication, or a room. Storyboards and diagrams explain how products work and how they fit into users' lives. Journey maps show how people can find their way through an architectural space or a digital interface.

A patient's history is an ongoing narrative. Diseases, procedures, treatments, and therapies are processes whose cause and effect demand understanding, which can be aided by diagrams and models as well as by words. Listening to a patient's own story—often muddled by electronic health records—is a crucial component of health care. The field of narrative medicine studies this area.

Storytelling takes place through every phase of health design thinking, from researching a problem to testing concepts and presenting them to others. User interviews invite stakeholders to tell stories while researchers listen for core insights. A persona is a hypothetical user, who—like a character in a novel—faces unique conflicts and has special skills and limitations. Maps and diagrams can show how a device functions, how a facility is used at different times of day, or how a disease spreads in a community. Role-playing with props and prototypes engages improv to quickly test concepts.

Storytelling is an essential tool for communicating health design concepts to others. A team at Thomas Jefferson University's Health Design Lab used sequential drawings to pitch their product FlipCatch, a device for collecting urine specimens. The team created drawings that range from friendly cartoons to technical diagrams, revealing both the functional and emotional stories that drive their product. Stories like these are as easy to understand as a comic strip.

Telling stories about a new medical device

Problem

These playful drawings introduce the problem addressed by FlipCatch, a product designed to collect clean midstream urine samples from women patients. These drawings show the current standard practice, a multistep process that requires patient training.

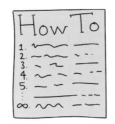

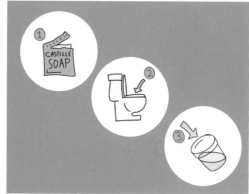

Emotion

These drawings show the difficulties caused by current methods. Collecting a clean sample with soap and water is awkward for patients and often results in contaminated samples.

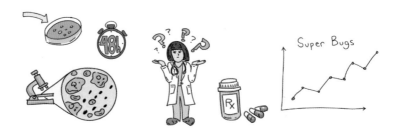

Solution

These technical drawings show how FlipCatch's internal mechanism isolates a sample of urine midstream, thereby preventing contamination.

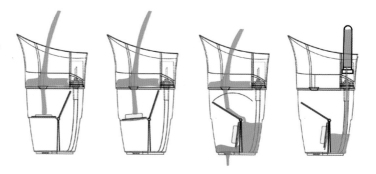

Design Team, Thomas Jefferson University: Anthony DiFranco, Christopher Neely, Dante Varotsis, and Helen Xu. Industrial design: 10xBeta

NARRATIVE ARC Novelists and screenwriters use the concept of the narrative arc to describe the rising and falling action of a typical story. In the beginning of the story, a problem is set forth. The action becomes more intense as the protagonist attempts to solve the problem (encountering and overcoming more obstacles along the way). The narrative arc rises and reaches a point of intensity—the climax—and then returns to a point of rest, leaving us with a satisfying sense of completion.

Telling a story with a sequence of pictures is an ancient concept. Instructions for using medical products are often depicted with sequential drawings, which can be understood across language and literacy levels. Filmmakers and designers often use storyboards to show action over time. A storyboard is both an exploratory tool for studying a problem and a means for communicating results. Effective storyboards depict a narrative with a beginning, a middle, and an end. (See Method | Storyboard.)

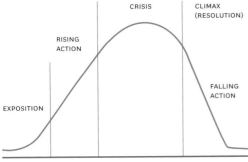

THE SHAPE OF STORIES Countless stories feature a pattern of rising and falling energy. Illustration adapted from Jack Hart, *Storycraft: The Complete Guide to Writing Narrative Nonfiction* (Chicago: University of Chicago Press, 2011).

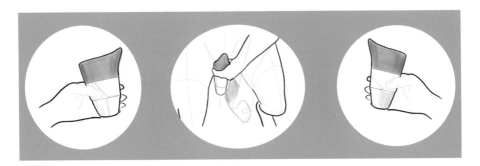

ONE, TWO, THREE Visual stories are often told in just a few panels. A sequence of three steps is easy to grasp and understand (beginning, middle, end). FlipCatch is a device for collecting clean urine samples.

INSTRUCTIONAL GRAPHICS A complex medical procedure or health care protocol has many steps. (Likewise, a novel or film has many scenes or chapters.) Each step can be broken down into smaller actions. Well-designed instructional graphics begin with careful analysis of the required steps. Are some parts of the procedure obvious? Do others require more details?

The visual timeline shown below was created by GoInvo, a design firm located in Boston, Massachusetts, specializing in creating services, systems, and information graphics for better health care. GoInvo created a visual guide that explains the personal protective equipment (PPE) health care workers must wear when treating patients with ebola. A sequence of simple icons helps workers to remember the main steps. More detailed drawings provide specific instructions, such as how to put on two pairs of gloves: one under the cuffs of the gown and one taped securely over the gown. A drawing of the full figure is annotated with numbers that are keyed to the timeline. An additional chart—with even more steps—shows how to remove the PPE.

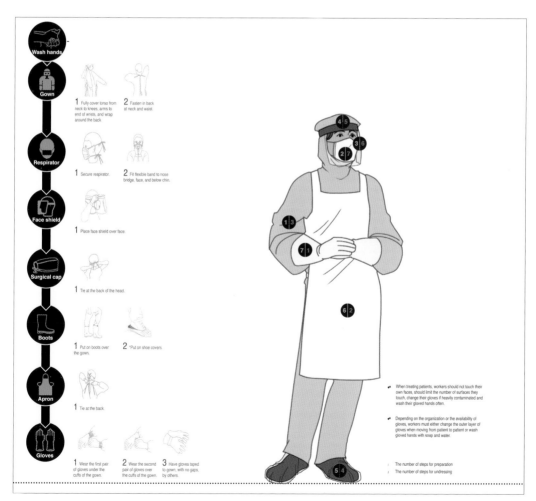

EBOLA CARE GUIDELINE (detail). Designed by GoInvo

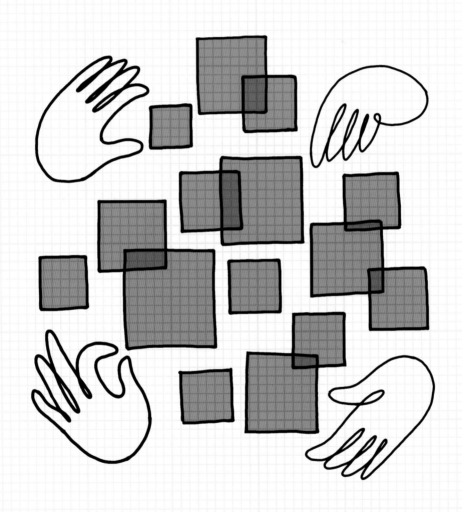

Methods

Around the world, patients, clinicians, and communities are beginning to apply the methods of design to health care problems. Many of the techniques presented here have been used for decades in fields such as advertising, product design, entrepreneurship, and social innovation, while others are uniquely suited to the health care space. Some design tools are easy to implement, while others require more time and expertise. No single method encompasses the entire design process. Design methods can be applied to brief immersive exercises or to extended projects.

Design Workshop

You can deliver a design workshop in a few hours, or you can spread it out over several days or an entire academic year. In the design workshops organized for medical students by the Health Design Lab at Thomas Jefferson University, health design faculty introduce dozens of design thinking methods to help future doctors become creative problem solvers in health care. Medical students who select the design track learn to think like designers by applying design methods to real challenges facing doctors.

Try running your own design workshop in addition to pursuing traditional approaches to researching a medical topic. A well-planned workshop can yield fresh insights. A workshop is a structured series of activities that primes people to think creatively, share ideas, and make those ideas concrete through project boards and simple prototypes. If you want to learn more about the latest therapies for managing asthma, invite people with asthma to a workshop in order to uncover unexpected concerns around inhaled steroids. If you are developing a plan to prevent thirty-day hospital readmissions in people with congestive heart failure (CHF), help your team crowdsource knowledge during a design workshop composed of diverse stakeholders, including clinicians, nurses, case managers, people with CHF, and caregivers.

A workshop alone will not be the basis of large-scale changes in an organization, but it can help open up people's minds to new thinking. Design workshops beat regular staff meetings for gaining deeper understanding of clinical problems and collecting authentic feedback. They can disrupt the business-as-usual mindset that locks down big institutions—especially hospitals. Workshops provide safe spaces for a wide range of stakeholders to become active participants in talking about a problem. Too often, a small group of "experts" dominates meetings; as a result, solutions are driven from the top down. Innovations in health care, however, come from all types of users. Listening to the stories of people who act as caregivers for their aging parents may inspire new ways to prevent hip fractures. Listening to elementary school kids can provide qualitative data to aid in designing hospitals that are less frightening for children.

To increase knowledge in a new area, run a design workshop with caregivers, families, and patients. Research can be fun!

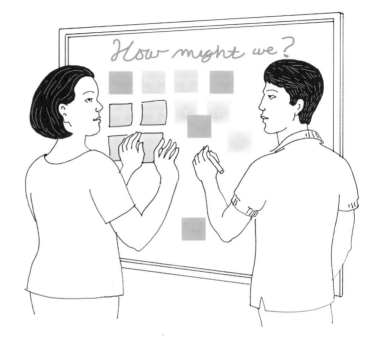

Planning a design workshop

Set the workshop challenge. Are you trying to improve a product, service, or space, or are you seeking new perspectives on a topic of concern?

Create an agenda. Include time for introductions, creative exploration, and sharing.

Set a time constraint. We suggest a minimum of 90 minutes.

Decide who to invite (minimum of 6 participants) and secure their participation.

Invite real users. For example, if you want to improve the registration process in a clinic, invite patients, receptionists, administrators, caregivers, medical assistants, nurses, and clinicians.

Interview patients or other stakeholders to gain insights from their expertise.

Identify a user whose experience you hope to improve. Is it the non-English-speaking patient who needs a translator during the registration process? Or is it the nurse who desires a better way to determine when someone is ready to be taken into a room?

Working individually or in pairs, develop simple prototypes.

Share insights and solutions.

PARTICIPATORY DESIGN The Health Design Lab at Thomas Jefferson University Hospital wanted to learn more about end-of-life issues. Performing an exhaustive literature search in medical journals is not the only way to gain new knowledge in medicine. The Lab held a workshop on the topic of death and dying and invited the public and hospital employees to participate. People from many backgrounds attended, including a rabbi, a priest, an architect, a woman who had recently lost her husband, a visiting student from Bangladesh, and a business school administrator.

Many people are uncomfortable discussing death. In medicine, the conversation around dying remains siloed within the palliative care community. Death is a life-defining event that happens to all humans—and dying may well represent one of life's greatest design challenges.

Adam Hayden, a father of three boys from Indiana with a graduate degree in philosophy, found out that he had glioblastoma, a highly aggressive brain cancer, at age 35. We asked Adam to record a five-minute video with his iPhone about his thoughts on death and how this diagnosis has affected his life. In Adam's honest and candid video, he shared, "It's important that we bring death out of the shadows of taboo." Showing his video to participants helped us undertand the experience of a person with a terminal illness. Empathy is the ability to recognize and share the mental states of others. Cultivating empathy is one ingredient of a successful design workshop.

In this participatory design session, attendees shared their own beliefs and experiences around the topic of dying. To get comfortable with discussing mortality, the group began by writing their own obituaries for the *New York Times*. Prompted with the question, "What are the problems around death and dying in America?" individuals wrote down their thoughts with Sharpie pens on sticky notes. They read their notes aloud within teams of five to seven participants and placed them on a whiteboard. The exercise allowed for everyone's insights to be grouped into different themes. The workshop uncovered diverse cultural perspectives about dying—even within a group of 30 participants. They desired to see death not just as a medical problem. One team pointed out the lack of education around death and mocked up a storyboard that described how a child-friendly curriculum could teach kids about the cycle of life and death.

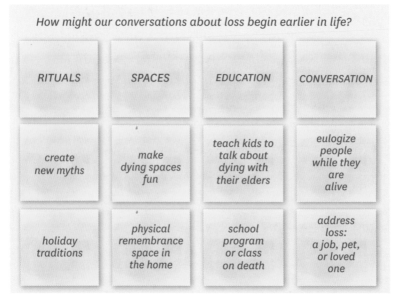

How might our conversations about loss begin earlier in life?

RITUALS	SPACES	EDUCATION	CONVERSATION
create new myths	make dying spaces fun	teach kids to talk about dying with their elders	eulogize people while they are alive
holiday traditions	physical remembrance space in the home	school program or class on death	address loss: a job, pet, or loved one

THINK AND SHARE Participants in a workshop can quickly generate ideas around different facets of a topic and organize them into groups.

Facilitating a group conversation

Breakout conversations can be planned as a part of a longer, multipart workshop.

Establish a time limit.

If group members don't know each other, make introductions. As an icebreaker, consider sharing something personal, such as favorite vacations.

A moderator can help ensure that everyone is heard within the allotted time.

A notetaker can collect insights and ideas.

Structure the conversation around a specific activity, such as creating a mind map, diagramming a process, or making a list of pros and cons.

Participants in a workshop about death and dying drafted their own obituaries for a future edition of a major newspaper.

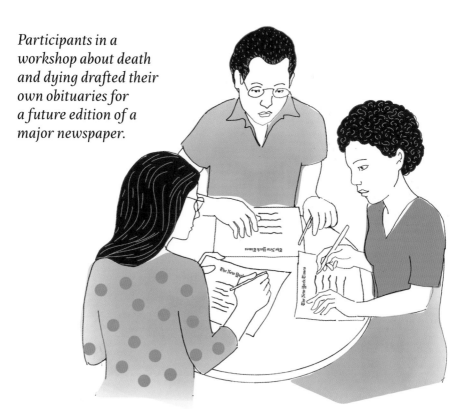

Brainstorming

Brainstorming was invented by advertising executive Alex Osborn in 1953. Osborn used this technique to help teams of people develop many creative concepts quickly, in a relaxed and uninhibited setting. The word "brainstorm" might make you think of a thundercloud raining down concepts. In fact, Osborn's metaphor isn't about the weather at all—it's from the military. A brainstorm bombards a single problem with ideas from every direction. Like a storm of bullets, most of these ideas will miss the mark, but a few may be worth developing further.

In a typical brainstorming session, a moderator asks the group for ideas and writes them down on sticky notes, a whiteboard, or a large pad of paper. The process can also be performed quietly, with everyone in the group writing down ideas before sharing them. This gives each team member a chance to think about the problem and develop insights. Starting with a period of independent work prevents any one person from dominating the session or setting the direction of the conversation at the outset.

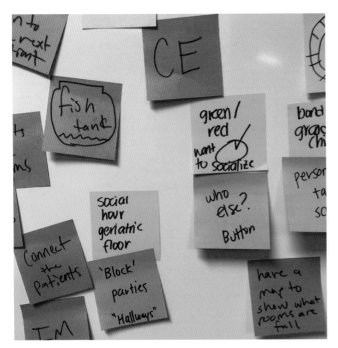

IDEAS, IDEAS, IDEAS Participants in a workshop led by the Health Design Lab at Thomas Jefferson University discussed ways to improve the mental health of older adults.

READ MORE Alex Osborn, *Applied Imagination: Principles and Procedures of Creative Thinking* (New York: Scribner, 1953).

Planning a brainstorming session

Establish a time limit. Participants will have more trust in the process if they know it won't be too long—anywhere from 15 to 45 minutes.

Define the goal or topic of the session. For example, before the group starts brainstorming, they could work together to define a "How might we..." question. Alternatively, the group organizer can begin the meeting with a clearly stated goal.

A moderator keeps time and makes sure everyone gets a chance to speak.

If possible, appoint a separate notetaker, who can concentrate fully on this task.

Write everything down. No one's ideas get rejected, no matter how strange or unlikely the proposals may be. Futuristic concepts can be the seed of viable products.

Reserve time for discussing the collected ideas. Sort them into categories to reveal patterns or trends. Combine and connect related concepts. Participants can use sticky dots to prioritize ideas for further development.

Don't just walk away from that wall of sticky notes. Do something with them! Transcribe them, photograph them, or collect them in a binder. Base an action plan on the session. Follow up with participants and share the results to keep them engaged in the process and let them know that their ideas are valuable and being acted on.

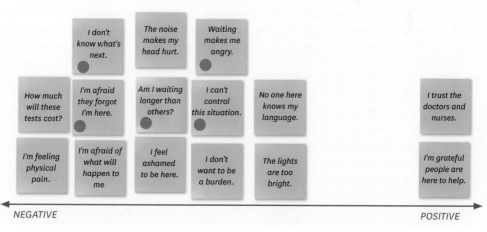

SORTING COMMENTS The simple process of sorting comments is an easy way to tap the power of visual thinking! Imagine that our research team has collected comments from patients in the ED. We sort the comments into positive and negative categories, which confirms the obvious: ED patients are anxious and uncomfortable. Yet the positive comments are significant, expressing trust and gratitude. The collected comments also confirm that waiting is a major source of distress for patients. Complaints about waiting are marked with red dots. Our team could decide to address patient distress about the experience of waiting, and the team could build on and amplify feelings of goodwill.

Interview

Interviewing patients and other users is one the most powerful tools in health design. Interviews yield insights into the motivations, goals, habits, fears, struggles, delights, and biases that influence human well-being. And patients—because of their unique experiences with addictions, injuries, physical pain, mental suffering, or life-ending illnesses—will have perspectives that are wildly divergent.

Interviews can reveal a person's mental model of a situation. For example, patients are often frustrated by long waits in the emergency department (ED). This experience can be especially vexing when others who arrive later are seen first by doctors. User interviews reveal that some people have the mental model of "first come, first served." This model may be applicable to waiting for a table at a restaurant—but it is not applicable to the ED. Breaking this rule violates people's expectations of fairness. Understanding this first come, first served mental model can help staff and clinicians seek better ways to communicate and lessen patients' frustration.

In an interview, power imbalances can make participants less forthright. Imagine a person talking to a doctor in a white coat, behind a desk, flanked by framed medical diplomas. Delivering negative feedback—already difficult for some people—can be even tougher when the interview subject is on the lower end of this power dynamic. Interviewers must take care to establish a safe and equal space. The interview subject is the teacher and expert—even if she is unemployed, is unhoused, and abuses substances.

While patients are the most important users, the provision of health care requires multiple participants—from doctors and nurses to friends and family. Different users may have conflicting needs. For example, even though patients are the primary users of hospital gowns, the gown must also interact with nurses and doctors in the setting of a physical examination, and with central supply workers, who must launder and maintain the gowns. While patients may desire more modest gowns—or to do away with such garments altogether—clinicians require ease of access and adequate exposure. Nearly any problem in health design requires interviewing users from diverse perspectives.

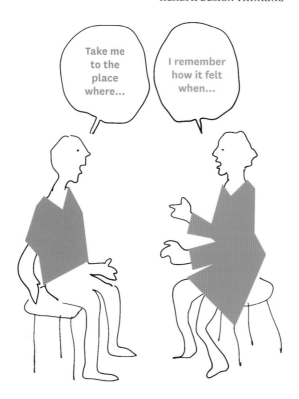

Starting a conversation

...and keeping it going

Tell me about...	...the transportation you used the last time you saw a doctor.
Describe the time when...	...you were brought into the hospital by ambulance.
Tell me the story of...	...the last time you were hospitalized.
Walk me through your experience of...	...the last time you took your family member to the hospital.
What was your best/worst...	...visit to an emergency room.

Begin with a phrase that lets your subject know that you care about their experience and genuinely want to learn about it.

Complete the question by inquiring about specific events rather than general concepts or judgments. The user is an expert in their own life story.

READ MORE Conversation openers come from Donald Norman, *The Design of Everyday Things* (New York: Basic Books, 2013), 244–45.

LIMITS OF THE INTERVIEW Understand what can go wrong in an interview. Users can mischaracterize the problem, misidentify the solution, or suffer from recall bias and faulty memory. People often emphasize daily annoyances over systemic problems. Ask a friend or colleague about their unmet needs—many will identify mundane problems rather than systemic failures. Such collective blind spots are why visions of the future often include housecleaning robots or flying cars. While Roombas have decreased the density of pet hair in our living spaces, they are trivial contributors to modern life.

In a complex system like health care, people have incomplete pictures of their own situations. A person might tell you that she felt scared coming to the hospital after a car crash but that the nurses were kind and she wished she could have seen the doctors more often. She might also tell you that because both her arms were casted, she had a hard time taking care of herself and felt a loss of dignity as she became dependent on others. What the person would not be able to tell you, however, was that her care was protocolized (often described as "trauma activation"), or that the trauma surgery team was understaffed, or that there was a shortage of nursing or medications. User predictions are notoriously poor, and their inferences about causality are limited. Thus, the most valuable user interviews focus on direct personal experiences and pain points.

User interviews in the context of health-related design face additional challenges. Most people have had some experience with pursuing health or seeking health care; these prior experiences can sometimes prevent us from fully empathizing with others. Good designers must actively unencumber themselves from preconceived notions. If you are already wearing a pair of shoes, it's hard to step into someone else's.

Asking better questions

Open-ended questions (rather than yes-no questions) help guide conversations more quickly to the portion of the experience most important to the user. The game Twenty Questions is funny and suspenseful because players have to guess what something is by asking only yes-or-no questions. That approach doesn't work in an interview, where you almost always want to ask questions that elicit specific, concrete details. In an interview, yes-no questions are vastly less interesting and effective.

Here's an open-ended way to start a conversation: "Walk me through your experience of going to the hospital after your car accident." Medical students are taught to begin taking patient histories by asking, "What brought you in today?" or "What can I do for you today?"

Once an area of interest is found, ask follow-up questions that probe for more details. Useful phrases include "You mentioned…" and "Please tell me more about…"

Uncover unmet needs with a hypothetical question: "If I had a magic wand that could fix one thing in your experience, which would you choose?"

Designers often use a technique called Five Whys to peel back layers of motivation. In this technique, each answer is met with another "Why?" in order to yield deeper insights about a topic.

Saying "I'm curious about…" or "Help me understand why…" can be less confrontational than just asking, "Why?" The tone will be perceived as less judgmental.

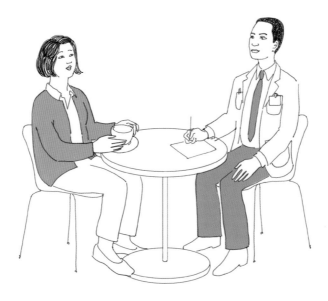

Conducting a user interview

Find a place that will feel comfortable and familiar to the interview subject. If appropriate, choose a location where the item or service being designed will be used. Will a device be used at home or in the hospital? The setting can yield additional insights. For example, a device that outputs auditory signals may not work well in a noisy practice location.

Create a psychologial space that is welcoming and safe. Frame the interview as a favor to the interviewer, and reassure the subject that the conversation will be nonjudgmental. Establish a power dynamic that respects the interview subject, placing them in the position of the teacher and expert.

As the interviewer, listen more than you talk. Slow down. Allow space for dead air. Don't rush to fill the pauses. Don't complete the other person's sentences. Give your subject time to answer. Practice pausing for ten seconds or more so that you can allow the interview subject to think and finish a thought. Practice with a stopwatch.

Bring a colleague to record the conversation so that you can pay full attention to your subject. If a colleague is not available, use a recording device. Making notes on paper is not ideal, but it is acceptable. Typing on laptops is distancing and distracting.

The fields of medicine and design use jargon and acronyms that are inaccessible to outsiders. Before sitting down with your users, have people outside of your field review your questions and point out problems. Answers gathered from interviews are one of the first outputs created in a health design project. Prototype and test your questions!

Photo Journal

If you are designing a product or service for a group of people—whether patients, health workers, or hospital administrators—understanding their stories in vivid detail can provide powerful clues to help you tailor your intervention. Using a photo journal is more helpful than working only with interviews for going more deeply into the everyday experiences of your target user.

To better understand what a "day in the life" looks like for the people most affected by your intervention, try asking a few users to make a simple photo journal that documents their daily routine. A project team at MICA's Center for Social Design worked with CAPABLE, a program created at the Johns Hopkins School of Nursing, to support teams of occupational therapists, nurses, and handypeople working with older adults in their homes. The team wanted to know what tools and skills helped the most successful frontline health workers do their jobs well. The goal was to help new trainees transition smoothly into the program. A photo journal was a valuable part of the process.

Asking potential users of a new product, service, or intervention to take a photo of "a few items in your bag—things you always keep with you" will reveal the tools of the trade that are important to users. Many of the visiting caregivers working with CAPABLE carry large bottles of hand sanitizer, clearly worn down from frequent use. Many of the photos in their photo journals were taken in the user's car.

What does this suggest about helping new CAPABLE team members achieve success? Ideas born of responses to these observations include leaving motivational messages or tips for new staff on items they use often, like hand sanitizer, or on places they'd see them often—like on an air freshener for their car. Short podcasts that caregivers could listen to between client visits might be more effective for ongoing training than written materials. The photo journal is not only a tremendously useful approach—it is also an enjoyable process for participants. Your team can use what you learn from photo journals to develop products and services that build on key user moments.

Creating a photo journal

PROMPTS Decide on a brief list of prompts for creating the journal. The ten photo prompts below relate to the tools and resources a traveling home care professional might use in a typical day. The last prompt asks for "anything else you want to show us from a typical day in your life," to keep the questions open-ended.

PICTURES Get snapping! Over the course of a day or a week, participants use their smartphones to capture photos as if they were on a scavenger hunt.

INTERPRETATION What do the photos mean? After participants submit their photos, it's time to study them. A tool called A.E.I.O.U.Y. (see page 71) is a useful checklist for observing and interpreting each image. This can be a stand-alone tool, or you can interview the participant after they've taken photos, asking them to walk you through the photos and talk about why they took each one.

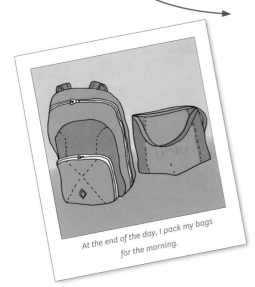

At the end of the day, I pack my bags for the morning.

PROMPTS FOR A PHOTO JOURNAL

- *The very start of your workday.*
- *The very end of your workday.*
- *A few items in your bag—things you always keep with you.*
- *A tool you find absolutely essential in your work.*
- *A moment that makes you feel frustrated.*
- *A moment that makes you feel happy.*
- *Someone you go to when you need a sounding board or advice.*
- *How you relax or recharge.*
- *Part of your job that makes you feel nervous, no matter how many times you do it.*
- *Anything else you want to show us from a typical day in your life.*

"Creating the photo journal was fun to do and the highlight of my day!"
PHOTO JOURNAL PARTICIPANT

hand
sanitizer

painter's
tape

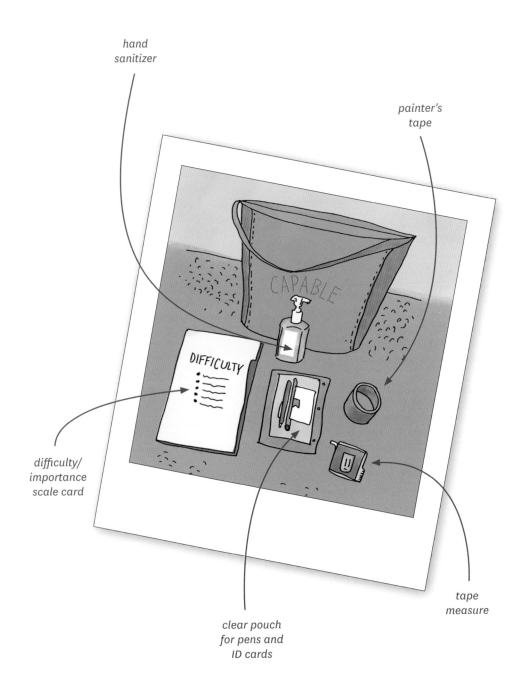

difficulty/
importance
scale card

tape
measure

clear pouch
for pens and
ID cards

A.E.I.O.U.Y. OBSERVATION CHART

	OBSERVATIONS	YOUR INTERPRETATION
ACTIVITIES What are people doing in this photo? What are their goals?	● Laying out bags the night before ● Staying organized ● Preparing for home visits	Like a plumber or electrician, a traveling home care professional brings their office with them.
ENVIRONMENTS Describe the space. Is it private? Shared? Comfortable? Sparse?	● No natural light—is it very late or very early? ● Plush carpeting; feels like the photo was taken at home	A home care professional's day starts and ends in their own home.
INTERACTIONS Between people and people? People and objects?	● No people-to-people interactions are shown in the photo	Solitary; the only person present appears to be the person taking the photo.
OBJECTS What objects, items, and tools do you see? How are they related to the activity going on?	● Tape measure for getting the correctly sized rugs ● Painter's tape for marking the house ● Hand sanitizer	Every item has a clear, practical function. Day-to-day work is mainly alone.
USERS Whom do you see? What do you know about them? How are they related? What are their roles?	● An occupational therapist, working in home care for senior citizens in Baltimore.	The careful presentation of the user's possessions for this photo indicates that they value staying organized.

Project team, MICA Center for Social Design: Ashley Eberhart, Faculty Advisor; Hannah Shaw, Community Liaison; Aditi Wagh, Anushka Jajodia, Cameron Morgan, Jess Sanders, and M Strickland, Design team. Partner: Johns Hopkins Center for Innovative Care in Aging: Sarah Szanton, Director; Sokha Koeuth, Program Manager; Janine Parisi, Advisor; Ally Evelyn Gustave, OT; Jill Roth, RN.

A.E.I.O.U.Y. Organize your thoughts around activities (A), environments (E), interactions (I), objects (O), users (U), and your interpretations (Y).

READ MORE On photo journals, → http://www.designkit.org/methods/65. On A.E.I.O.U.Y. charts, → https://help.ethnohub.com/guide/aeiou-framework

Persona

A persona is a fictional character who represents potential users. Each persona is identified with a visual portrait and a background narrative. Each persona has a name, allowing the design team to talk about them during the design process. For example, "Jane will need room here for her wheelchair," or "Carlos will be with his grandmother." Personas are archetypal individuals, who help designers see a new product, service, or experience from the perspectives of users. The most effective personas are based on interviews and observations conducted with real individuals. Because they are free of stereotypes, personas highlight the deeper motivations, frustrations, and adaptations of human beings.

Developing personas takes time and creativity. The goal is to bring each persona to life with a concise set of narrative details relevant to the design challenge at hand. Crafting an inclusive group of personas is critical. Beyond including the typical or "average" user of a product or service, the design team should seek to identify outliers—or what the design consulting firm IDEO calls "extreme users." These outliers include novice and expert users of a service as well as people with diverse abilities and cultural backgrounds. The process of creating a set of personas derived from a wide range of user experiences can help designers unlock new approaches and insights.

Participating in the UVA Medical Design Program at the University of Virginia School of Medicine (UVA), a cohort of first-year medical students used human-centered design approaches to explore ways to improve patient experience in the ED. In particular, the students focused on enhancing the design and operation of public spaces in the ED, such as the entry lobby and waiting areas. The project was timely for the UVA health system, given the concurrent design and construction of a new emergency and critical care facility.

The project resulted in a set of posters describing different users of the ED. Every user brings unique needs and desires to the task of waiting for medical care. Personas illustrate these diverse goals and capacities and make them present to the design team and other decision makers.

Creating a user persona

Developing a user persona is like creating a character for a novel. The persona has abilities, limitations, and goals—and a life beyond the context of your design challenge. You can make a product or service more delightful and inclusive by drawing on the wisdom of each persona. Building on experience and intuition and on user interviews and observations, the design team creates a set of personas who represent a range of possible users. After building a narrative around each persona, the team makes a set of posters. These posters guide the design process.

NAME Pick a name that is easy to remember. Use this name in conversations about the design challenge: "What would Ashley do here?"

BACKSTORY Name some defining events in this character's life. She could be a person who does not speak English or a college student whose family is far away.

SCENARIO Create a short narrative sketch in which the persona confronts a challenge. What situation has brought her to the hospital or clinic today?

EMOTIONS How does the persona feel about her situation? Is she confident, overwhelmed, or angry? What emotions are her caregivers expressing?

MOTIVATION What does the persona want to achieve? Is she seeking attention for a sudden crisis or a chronic condition?

BEHAVIORS What is the persona doing to achieve her goals? Is a family member assisting in the process? What pressures is the caregiver responding to?

ABILITY INHIBITORS What actions or situations—such as physical pain, a concerned relative, or a language barrier—might be causing anxiety or distress?

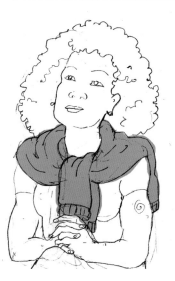

SCENARIO *Miranda is a single mother with diabetes. She needs emergency care for diabetic ketoacidosis (DKA). Miranda is worried about waiting because her young children are staying with a neighbor who needs to leave for work. She is a frequent visitor to the ED and knows some of the staff by name.*

PRIORITIZING THE PATIENT Emergency departments are often chaotic, unnerving, and frustrating environments for people—particularly those with urgent but not life-threatening needs. Most critical care environments cater primarily to the needs of clinicians, heavily prioritizing the process-oriented demands of health care. Although this approach may be justifiable in the context of true medical emergencies, many people depend on the ED as an access point for urgent yet non-life-threatening medical issues. The utilitarian character of ED facilities and customer service delivery can make the experience for these patients and their caregivers unnecessarily harsh and impersonal.

The medical students started by analyzing clinical databases to understand the overall distribution of ED patients, as traditionally defined by demographic and medical encounter data, in the UVA ED. Next, they conducted interviews with key stakeholders (nurses, techs, receptionists, physicians) to identify groups whose medical needs, comfort requirements, and other considerations were not well addressed. Examples included elderly individuals, people in wheelchairs, individuals requiring pain control (such as adults with migraines and children with sickle cell anemia), and patients needing to make frequent visits to the ED for unscheduled treatment of longer-term complex conditions (such as chemotherapy infusion).

Working together, the medical students used insights from their secondary research to create a preliminary set of proto-personas. A proto-persona is a working draft of potential patient groups to highlight, based on accumulated anecdotes and researchers' intuition.

This work helped the team organize and focus their goals and strategies for their primary data collection efforts.

Over the next several weeks, each student conducted research shifts in the ED waiting room, seeking to better understand the experience of patients and families. The students captured their observations using a variety of structured research approaches. For qualitative observations, they used a framing tool called "I Noticed, I Wonder," which helps researchers observe and record behaviors without applying their own biased interpretations. The students also conducted five-minute quantitative tallies of observed behaviors in the various ED public spaces; they noted how patients and their caregivers used and inhabited the ED's public spaces while waiting to be placed in a clinical care room.

After completing their own primary research in the ED, the medical students met for a final workshop to synthesize their data and create a first set of UVA ED patient personas. The students focused on people's shared challenges and behaviors, rather than on demographics or medical conditions, to delineate differences in needs and desires during initial phases of an ED visit. For example, multiple students were surprised to see how many people required a wheelchair in the waiting room. This not only made the seating areas crowded but also made it difficult for these patients and their caregivers to sit together.

At the conclusion of the workshop, the medical students translated their insights into large-format posters depicting several personas and narratives. These personas were used throughout the remainder of the semester to inform the students' service design projects in the ED.

READ MORE On extreme users, see Ideo.org, *The Field Guide to Human-Centered Design*, → www.designkit.org/methods/45. On personas, see Christoph Zürn, "The Persona Core Poster," Creative Companion (2011), → www.creativecompanion.wordpress. com/2011/05/05/the-persona-core-poster/; and Alan Cooper, "The Origin of Personas," Cooper.com (2008), → www.cooper.com/journal/2017/4/the_origin_of_personas

DIFFERENT USERS Creating personas for users of the UVA ED offered students in the medical design program an introduction to both design thinking and the challenges faced by patients and caregivers. Development of research-based personas also yielded an important new resource at UVA—a simple tool for incorporating patient perspectives into wide-ranging decisions about the design and operation of the new ED.

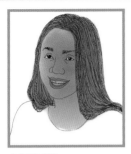

ASHLEY

A young expert patient in a new town

17-year-old woman with migraines arrives at the ED with acute onset of a severe headache. She is new to town, having just started undergrad at UVA. She is a highly informed patient with a detailed care plan but has been receiving care from a team at her hometown hospital in California. Her parents, who are very involved in her care, have already called the ED to check on her.

"I wish I could talk to my doctor back home. And I wish my mom and dad were here now…"—ASHLEY

MOTIVATION

ASHLEY wants the pain to stop. She wants to go home, where she can get away from the bright lights and loud noises of the ED.

MOM & DAD want Ashley's physician at her hometown hospital to call all the shots and tell UVA's ED what to do.

BEHAVIORS

ASHLEY is tired of telling her medical history to multiple people (triage nurses, techs, medical students, residents, attending physicians). She asks if they can just get her medical records from home already.

MOM & DAD are texting and FaceTiming Ashley constantly and asking to speak to ED staff every 20 minutes to ask what's going on and make suggestions.

ABILITY INHIBITORS

ASHLEY is having a hard time keeping her composure because her headache is so severe. She is getting impatient with her parents and with the clinical care team.

MOM & DAD are upset that they're not physically present with their daughter.

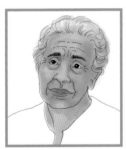

SUE

A recent immigrant with a ground-level fall

60-year-old woman who speaks only Tibetan is brought to the ED by her neighbor Jane, who saw her fall in her driveway. The patient is holding her hip. The patient's daughter is on her way to the hospital but is traveling from far away and won't arrive for a few hours.

"I really wish I could talk to my daughter."—SUE

MOTIVATION

SUE wants to communicate with the care team, but no one speaks her language.

JANE, Sue's neighbor, wants to help Sue but doesn't know how to communicate very well with her.

BEHAVIORS

SUE is trying to talk to the ED team and to Jane in Tibetan. A lot of people are saying things to Sue in English, and this seems to make her more upset as time goes on.

JANE is trying to help Sue use Google Translate on her phone to communicate with her and with the ED team.

ABILITY INHIBITORS

SUE is in pain, not sure what's going to happen to her, and very concerned about getting an expensive bill from the hospital.

JANE wants to help her neighbor and doesn't want to leave her alone without a translator, but she is supposed to be at a family gathering and needs to leave before Sue's daughter arrives.

Creating a poster for each persona— and keeping it visible in the work area—helps a design team focus on human needs, not just on technical outcomes.

Role-Playing

Role-playing is a form of experiential prototyping. Using minimal props, participants act out the interactions involved in delivering a service, using a device, or completing a procedure. The process of physically running through a scenario can help a design team optimize the elements of a doctor–patient interaction or troubleshoot awkward moments in the use of a device.

A patient exam can be improvised with name tags, a white coat, and a fake cough. A makeshift exam table can be made by covering a desk with white butcher paper. A monitor showing a patient's chest X-ray can be mocked up with a simple sketch taped to a wall. Rough prototypes or 3D-printed models of diagnostic devices can be tried out for size with patients and clinicians.

Role-playing can be used to uncover problems with existing products and practices and to test new ideas. Designers, patients, and clinicians can all take part in role-playing exercises. Swapping roles helps participants build empathy with each other. Role-playing is fast, cheap, and often illuminating.

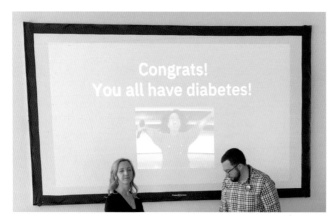

CONGRATS! YOU ALL HAVE DIABETES!
The Health Design Lab at Thomas Jefferon University led an all-staff workshop for IMRE, a company that develops marketing and advertising for health care products. Workshop leaders Kristy Shine (left) and Rob Pugliese (right) enacted a scene in which a physician delivers a diabetes diagnosis to a patient. Playing the role of doctor, Pugliese overwhelmed his "patient" with information about the medications, procedures, and risks that this patient would immediately become responsible for. Workshop participants were asked to imagine themselves receiving the same news. This powerful role-playing exercise primed the group to develop ideas for improving the health of patients grappling with a new diagnosis.

SHARING RESULTS Radiation oncology residents at Thomas Jefferson University are prototyping a mobile app that allows access to a patient's treatment regimen and addresses patient concerns such as side effects. The residents have created an oversized cardboard mock-up of a digital tablet. Interacting with this improvised device is a physical activity that engages the whole team.

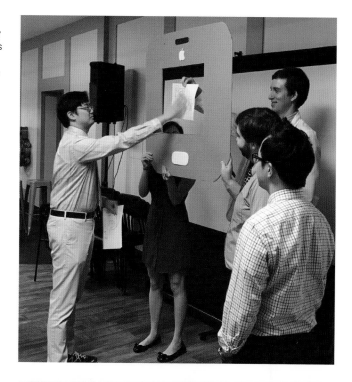

WHO'S IN THE ROOM? Medical students at Thomas Jefferson University are addressing the confusion and discomfort patients feel when they don't know the roles of all the people entering their patient room. During a hospital encounter, a patient interacts with a changing roster of people who are directly or indirectly involved in their care—nurses, technicians, resident physicians, social workers, support staff, and medical students. It's challenging for patients to recognize these people and understand what role they perform. The proposed solution, initially sketched on a whiteboard, incorporates a digital screen displaying a photo and a description of a patient's care team. The students in this exercise are acting out the proposed solution.

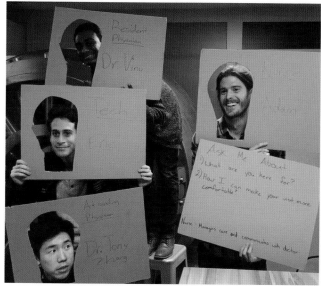

Role Cards

Design thinking works best when the process inspires a group of people to imagine new possibilities instead of falling back on old ways of working ("We've tried that before" or "That's just the way things work around here"). In health care, people are trained to have tightly defined roles and responsibilities. Although this training helps us to deliver safe and effective care, it can stifle imagination when we want to take creative risks.

Role cards are a tool for developing the creative mindset. This quick exercise can help break down social hierarchies and static world views by encouraging people to take on a creative task or a leadership position they might not otherwise adopt. This technique works both in a one-time session and in a long-term task force.

Building trust and autonomy in interdisciplinary groups takes conscious effort, but it pays off in the quality of collaboration and ideas. If you like this method, take a look at Edward de Bono's *Six Thinking Hats* and the School of Life's *100 Questions: Work Edition*. These books contain mind-opening ideas for helping members of a team work together and keep each other's goals in mind.

Making and using role cards

1. PREPARE Before starting a design challenge, take a set of index cards and write the name of one role on each card. Ideally, you want as many roles as you have people. In smaller teams, some participants may double up.

2. SET ROLES When planning the first meeting of a design thinking group, block off time to discuss team roles. Explain each of the roles to your team and ask if there are any other roles that should be added.

3. DRAW CARDS Next, everyone randomly draws a card and announces the role that they will play. To build excitement and a sense of playfulness, ask the room for a drumroll, or play the theme song from *2001: A Space Odyssey* (no, really).

4. REPEAT Decide how often you want people to switch roles. For example, if the team meets once a month, members might draw cards at each meeting and play their new roles during the meeting and throughout the month to come.

READ MORE David M. Kelley and Tom Kelley, *Creative Confidence: Unleashing the Creative Potential Within Us All* (New York: Random House, 2013); → www.scottjeffrey.com/six-thinking-hats/; → www.theschooloflife.com/shop/us/100-questions-work-edition/

Suggested team roles

THE USERS' ADVOCATE Your job is to nudge us to link our ideas to what we have heard from real people.

THE VISUALIZER You will help draw system maps, diagrams, and other visual representations.

THE DOCUMENTER You will capture key points and ideas. Write notes, take photos, record share-outs, and make sure we all have access to these resources afterwards.

THE DREAMER Put your head in the clouds: imagine what we'd do if we could rock the whole system.

THE FACILITATOR Ensure everyone's voice is heard. Gently push and support the group, floating among breakouts.

THE RESEARCHER Point out real-world situations. Support theory with observation. Question the group's assumptions.

THE MANAGER Your task...is to keep us on task. Anytime someone names an action item, write it down. Ask, "How will we make that happen?"

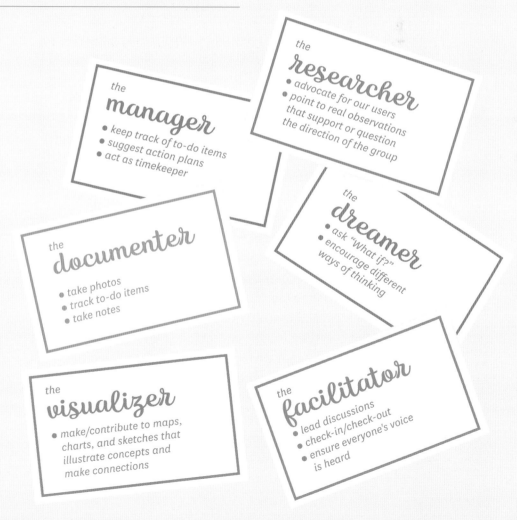

the **researcher**
- advocate for our users
- point to real observations that support or question the direction of the group

the **manager**
- keep track of to-do items
- suggest action plans
- act as timekeeper

the **dreamer**
- ask "what if?"
- encourage different ways of thinking

the **documenter**
- take photos
- track to-do items
- take notes

the **visualizer**
- make/contribute to maps, charts, and sketches that illustrate concepts and make connections

the **facilitator**
- lead discussions
- check-in/check-out
- ensure everyone's voice is heard

Storyboard

Comic books and graphic novels are popular forms of literature around the world. People of all ages enjoy and understand stories told in the comic book format: a series of images in chronological order, annotated with speech bubbles and thought clouds.

A storyboard consists of a few pictures or sketches with notes that explain the action. Filmmakers use storyboards to plan the visual flow of a movie. Designers use them to plan the interactive use of a product or service.

A storyboard explains action primarily through visual images. A few simple drawings can be "read" more quickly than a hefty paragraph of text. An adage posted on the walls of countless high school writing classrooms warns young writers, "Show, don't tell." Storyboards help us show action, purpose, and emotion. The images in a storyboard can be drawn by hand or photographed. In a workshop setting, participants can sketch on sheets of paper that have been pre-printed with four to six boxes.

To plan a storyboard, you will need to decide what action you are trying to convey and how to represent that action in just a few frames. The first frame of a storyboard sets the scene. Where are we? What is the problem or situation? You might also decide at the outset how the story will end and then fill in the steps needed to get there. Alternatively, the process of sketching a storyboard can be more open-ended, becoming a tool for finding an answer or solution.

Powerful stories show characters and action. The characters have a problem they want to solve or a task they need to complete, such as enrolling patients in a clinical trial or getting to a medical appointment. An effective storyboard shows an action from beginning to middle to end. It depicts objects and details that are necessary to the story, but nothing else. Learning to tell a story in a few simple frames will help you convey ideas quickly to others and focus on the elements of action, transformation, and emotional impact that drive effective design concepts.

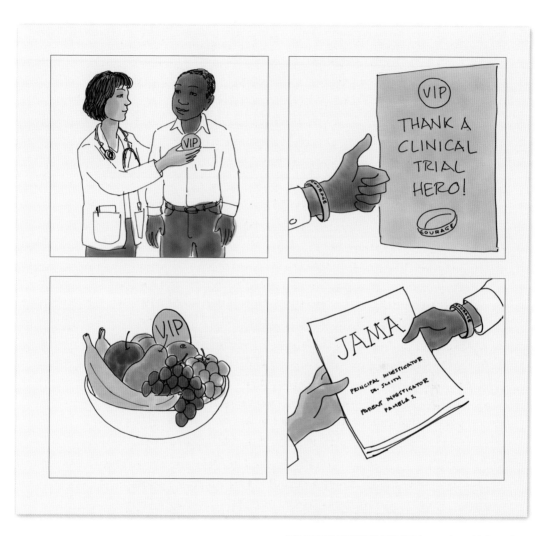

CREATING STORYBOARDS This storyboard is based on a sketch from a workshop led by the Health Design Lab at Thomas Jefferson University, where patients reported that they did not feel recognized for their efforts in participating in clinical trials. Creating storyboards is a useful tool for generating and shaping ideas and for sharing diverse perspectives on a topic.

Using storyboards to develop ideas

Storyboards are valuable throughout the design process, from early workshops (when diverse participants are generating ideas) to farther downstream (when teams are pitching concepts to investors or stakeholders).

Pre-printed templates can be helpful. You can find templates online or make your own. Four to six frames is a good number for a design workshop. (Storyboards for filmmakers will have many more panels.)

For team work, standard copy paper may be too small. Use a ruler to divide a large sheet of paper into frames. A team can gather around the sheet to work, or it can be easily shared with a larger group.

Use drawings of people and simple dialogue to depict an emotional situation, not just a technical solution. Don't worry about how well you draw. Stick figures are an ancient and universal expression of the human condition!

Storyboard

SCENARIO	PRODUCT OR SERVICE
Anne has complex new dietary restrictions	*Meal delivery service*

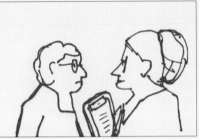

Anne and her doctor discuss Anne's new dietary restrictions and how the plan will work. Anne is worried.

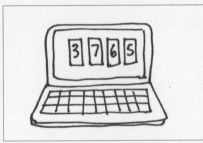

Anne enters a code on her computer that specifies her new food restrictions. It's easy!

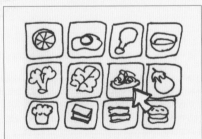

Anne chooses her first week of meals from a menu of options. There are many choices.

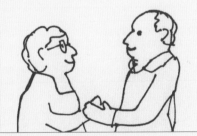

A delivery technician arrives with frozen meals. He talks with Anne and asks how she is doing.

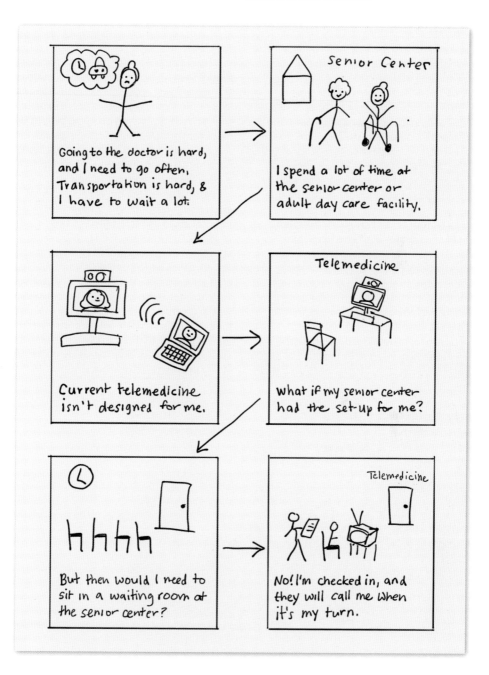

PROBLEMS AND SOLUTIONS These storyboards (opposite and above) are based on sketches created in workshops organized by the Health Design Lab, Thomas Jefferson University. A storyboard can be four panels, six panels, or more.

STORY OF SELF Storytelling is a valuable tool for helping clinicians and medical staff communicate the value of their work. Organizations and social movements around the world use a concept called "public narrative" to tap into not just what they do, but why they do it and how to move others to action. Developed by community organizer and scholar Marshall Ganz, the first part of this public narrative framework is developing a Story of Self— identifying a personal story that describes "why you were called to what you have been called to."

Patient safety is a branch of health care that focuses on ending preventable medical error. Building a culture of safety requires trust and communication among clinicians, staff, and patients. The Center for Social Design at the Maryland Institute College of Art (MICA) teamed up with Johns Hopkins Medicine's Armstrong Institute for Patient Safety and Quality to understand how storytelling might encourage clinicians to talk about patient safety.

The design team developed an interactive booklet and activity inspired by the Story of Self to help people tell the story of what motivated them to help build a culture of safety at their hospital. To test the concept, they shared their stories in a small group workshop. A nurse recounted a story from when she was a trainee, curious about observing opportunities to improve care in her unit. A manager talked about experiences she had recently had with helping people feel more comfortable during tense, stressful times. As participants shared their individual stories, patterns emerged that told a bigger story about their collective vision and values.

Participants in the project also brainstormed ideas for how patient safety advocates in any hospital could use storytelling to build a culture of safety. One idea was for a pop-up storytelling space featuring story prompts and games that a department's patient safety liaison could use to start conversations during advocacy events like Patient Safety Awareness Week. Another concept was to create a guided tour through the hospital for a new patient safety liaison's first day on the job—with "stops" along the way to hear true stories about times when speaking up for patient safety made a positive impact.

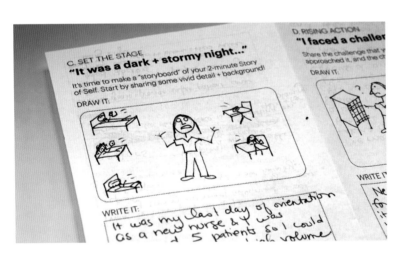

TELL YOUR OWN STORY Participants in this storytelling workshop began by brainstorming situations where they encountered challenges. They chose one example to narrate more fully.

MICA Center for Social Design: Ashley K. Eberhart, Design Lead. Armstrong Institute for Patient Safety and Quality, Johns Hopkins Medicine: Eileen Kasda, Project Advisor; Mike DiJulia, Partnership Lead; Christine Robson, Collaborator

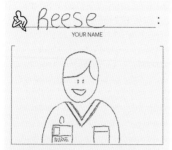

Reese :
YOUR NAME

STORY OF SELF

Build a story that engages + inspires

A. GIVE YOUR STORY A PURPOSE.
Consider your goals + audience.

1. What is **one change** that you personally want to make through your work?

Support other nurses to act on their ideas!

2. Name **one specific audience** that you have trouble explaining your work (or the value of your work) to.

my mentees

3. What **values** do you think this audience holds? What **goals** do they have that may be similar to yours?

Wanting to give the best care to patients. Feeling valued. Growing.

B. CONNECT YOUR GOAL TO YOUR VALUES.
Choose a personal story to tell.

4. **What story can you tell about your life** that would reveal that you have similar values to the audience and explain to them why you are called to leadership on your issue?

Take 2 minutes to brainstorm as many ideas as you can. Ready? **Circle your top choice.**

nursing school trip to Honduras

my first promotion

(fall prevention initiative)

advice my mom gave me

caring for patient with dementia   NOW, OPEN ME!

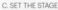

Standard office paper, printed on both sides, folded in half and in half again to make a small booklet

C. SET THE STAGE
"It was a dark + stormy night..."

It's time to make a "storyboard" of your 2-minute Story of Self. Start by sharing some vivid detail + background!

DRAW IT:

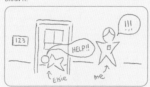

WRITE IT:

Never forget first patient fall
- Elsie, recovering from stroke, wanted to go home in time for grandson's birthday
- Her face crumpled in pain, frustrated

D. RISING ACTION
"I faced a challenge..."

Share the challenge that you faced, how you approached it, and the choice that you made.

DRAW IT:

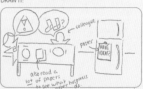

WRITE IT:

I wondered how many patients like Elsie were out there. Was nervous about speaking up, so I started with brainstorms in the lunch room, and asking patients

E. FALLING ACTION
"From that day forward..."

Share the outcome of your choice, and how it led to you becoming a patient safety advocate.

DRAW IT:

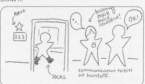

WRITE IT:

Got simple tricks approved, like red nonslip socks, that patients said made them feel safer without embarrassing them. Made a big difference!

F. SHARE THE MEANING
"That's why you should..."

Connect it all back to the values that you share with your audience and the action(s) you want them to take.

DRAW IT:

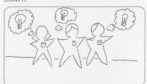

WRITE IT:

I learned that we have the tools within us to be creative and design solutions that make patients safer, and help us grow as nurses. What's _your_ idea?

STORY BUILDER This sample story was created to demonstrate the use of the template. You can download a ready-to-use version of this tool:
→ www.bit.ly/healthcarestoryofself

GRAPHIC MEDICINE Comics are more than just stories about superheroes or entertainment for kids. Clinicians have used comics to share personal experiences and emotions from a fresh perspective. Patients and caregivers have used comics to express their own narratives about living with a mental illness or caring for a dying parent.

The term "graphic medicine" is widely used in reference to comics serving as a medium for visual storytelling in health care. The term was coined by Ian Williams, MD, a physician and comic artist. Graphic stories have become accepted as a legitimate medium for patient care and medical education. Medical journals including the *Annals of Internal Medicine* and *AMA Journal of Ethics* publish comics alongside traditional text-heavy research studies.

A comic is a type of storyboard that typically is intended as its own form of communication rather than as a plan for another work. In a health design thinking workshop, participants can use comics to convey personal narratives, express the emotional side of a design challenge, or tell the story of a persona or user.

Comics can communicate action and insights more efficiently than a page full of text. They are a good format for communicating health information about diseases or delivering instructions for medical procedures. A child undergoing a procedure may be less frightened after reading a comic showing what to expect. A doctor might be more willing to share her experiences of grief, anxiety, and joy in health care through a graphic story than through a personal essay.

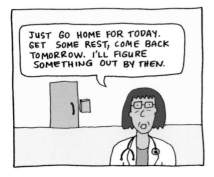

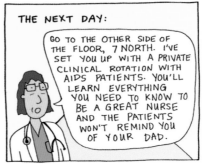

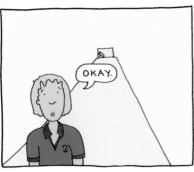

NURSE'S PERSPECTIVE *Taking Turns: Stories from HIV/AIDS Care Unit 371* is a graphic novel by MK Czerwiec. The book combines her memories with the oral histories of patients, family members, and staff. She depicts life and death on the ward, the ways the unit was affected by those who passed through it, and how many look back on their time there today.
© 2017 MK Czerwiec

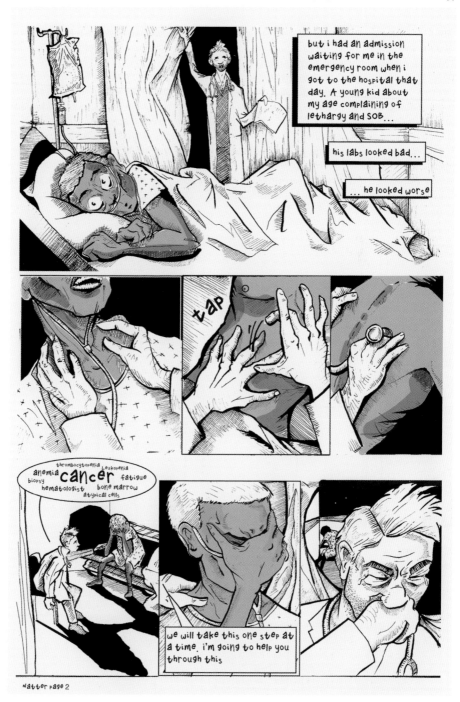

Mike Natter, MD, "Progress Notes: Cancer," Annals of Internal Medicine 170 (2019): W73–W77.

DESIGNING DIGITAL PRODUCTS Storyboards are crucial tools for developing digital products. Today, numerous apps help people monitor their own care in addition to connecting them with information, patient communities, and medical professionals. Such apps—which could extend access to health care—are a major opportunity for design thinking and innovation.

The design firm GoInvo specializes in creating apps and information systems for health care. Unlike watching a movie, using an app is a nonlinear experience. Users make choices and find their own way through different types of content and different modes of interaction. Storyboards are one of the tools designers use to plan these interactions. A single app may support many different experiences—from responding to a chatbot or having a live conversation with a doctor to tracking medications. Sequential screen designs help bring these interactions to life. Designers use prototyping software to create interactive versions of their initial sketches or wireframe drawings, which allows them to simulate the experience of the final app before it is developed.

1. HOMESCREEN

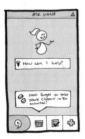

2. DANA, PERSONAL HEALTH ASSISTANT

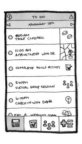 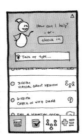

3. GROUP SESSIONS

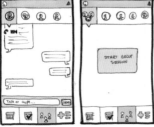 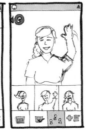

4. EDUCATION GOALS

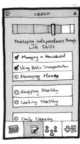 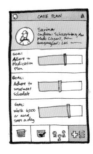

5. HEALTH METRICS

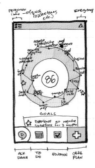 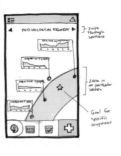

6. HEALTH STATUS SENSING AVATAR

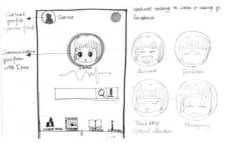

HUMAN-COMPUTER INTERACTION A digital app is more than a collection of screen designs. It is a complex system accessed by humans and machines working across different networks. Software designers and systems engineers create diagrams to document and explain information systems. A network for storing and retrieving patient records has numerous nodes, including medical workers, patients, computer terminals, and databases housed at different hospitals. Along the way, decisions are made by living people and by automated processes.

Designers at GoInvo use storytelling to make complex systems and workflows understandable. To show how a health records system will be used, they created a scenario and described each step of the process. Adding pictures makes the scenario more concrete and relatable. Numbered captions guide readers through the story. Arrows connecting the pictures emphasize relationships and clarify the narrative action. Including people in the drawings brings home the fact that digital products are ultimately created by and for human beings.

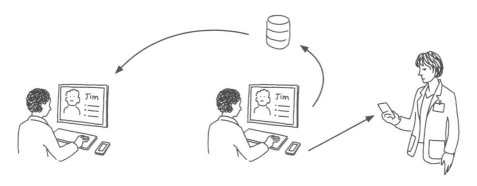

Data-consented patient information is displayed to the specific provider. Medications, allergies, and contraindications are automatically consented data. Other data elements are not. The displayed information has been pulled from the hospital's SHR database.

The PCP logs new information directly into the patient's SHR, which is automatically translated into a standardized format and housed within the hospital's SHR database.

The PCP sends a direct or SFTP patient referral message to a specialist at a neighboring hospital. Patient consents the specialist to view the SHR.

MENTAL HEALTH (left) These screen designs represent a digital app for patients with schizophrenia. This complex app includes a calendar for self care, video group sessions, medication tracking, patient education, and overall health metrics. More complex features are explained with multiple screens. Design: GoInvo

DATA ACCESS WORKFLOW (above; detail, redrawn) Sequential images and text show how an electronic Health Information Exchange (HIE) will be used. In this scenario, a primary care physician sends new patient information to the HIE and then refers a patient to a specialist. Design: GoInvo

Making a photo-based storyboard

Storyboards can be created with photographs instead of drawings. A photo-based storyboard shown within a presentation deck feels vivid and real—but producing it is far easier than shooting and editing a video.

After planning your action, assemble your actors in an appropriate setting. Use props or prototypes to represent your product. Shoot lots of pictures, and pick the best ones to tell the story.

If you are prototyping a digital app, use Photoshop to add screen designs to your pictures. Speech bubbles and descriptive text can be added with Powerpoint or other presentation software.

Design: GoInvo

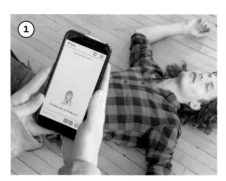

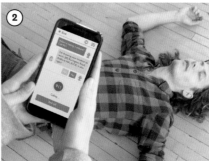

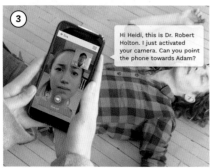

Hi Heidi, this is Dr. Robert Holton. I just activated your camera. Can you point the phone towards Adam?

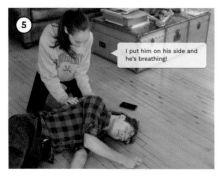

Please put Adam on his side

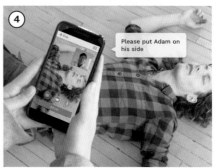

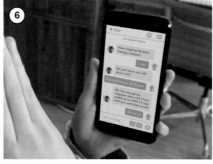

I put him on his side and he's breathing!

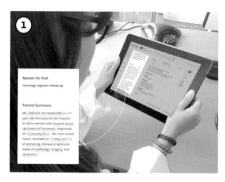

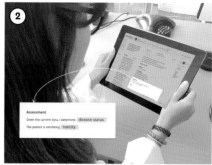

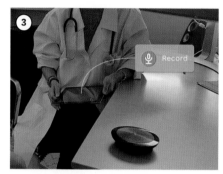

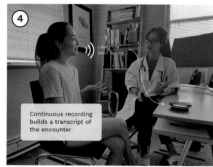

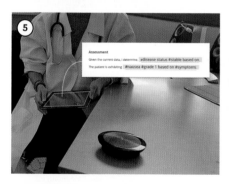

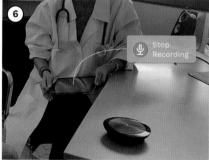

Continuous recording builds a transcript of the encounter

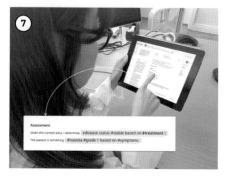

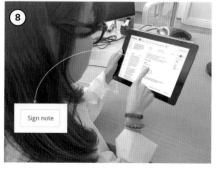

Journey Map

Journey maps help us understand a user's experience of a product, service, or space over time. Architects use journey maps to analyze existing health care facilities. How do patients find services inside a hospital? How do nurses gather the supplies needed for procedures? What barriers stand in their way? Spatial data maps are made by observing how people move around a facility and by interviewing them about their journeys. Maps can be made by a team discussing a floor plan and making notes on it.

Many journey maps represent a process rather than a physical space. Designers use journey maps to imagine a user's interaction with a device or service or to break down the components of a current offering. The journey map on the opposite page was created during a health design workshop in which participants developed blue-sky or visionary product concepts for patients newly diagnosed with type 2 diabetes. Participants used a template to show a treatment device being introduced to a patient. The journey map shows multiple layers of the user's experience, such as the action taking place and the emotional response to the situation.

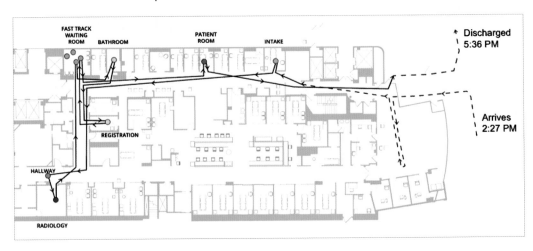

NAVIGATING THE ED This map was made by observing a single patient who was seen and discharged in the fast-track area of an emergency department. It was created as a part of a larger study of space use in the ED. Design: KieranTimberlake

Journey Map

	Scenario	User goals	Product or service
	Sarah is newly diagnosed with T2 diabetes.	*Sarah wants to tackle her new normal.*	*Embracelet—diabetes treatment hub*

Stages

Diagnosis	*Sarah receives tool for customizing treatment.*	*Sarah prioritizes immediate needs.*	*Sarah and her doctor stay informed.*

Action | What is the user doing?

Sarah receives the news of her type 2 diabetes diagnosis from her doctor.	*She puts on the Embracelet and syncs it to the platform.*	*Manage appointments, get reminders for refills, send vitals to clinicians, tap the bracelet for info, and communicate with care team.*	*Sarah shares info with her care team. They can support her when she needs help.*

Touchpoints | How does the user interact with the product or service?

Emotion | What is the user thinking and feeling?

Overwhelmed. Sarah is consumed with negative emotions. She feels paralyzed.	*Skeptical. Will this really help?*	*Comforted. Her condition begins to feel more manageable.*	*Confident. Sarah will be able to handle this.*

WEARABLE TREATMENT HUB This journey map is based on sketches created during a workshop led by the Health Design Lab at Thomas Jefferson University with employees at IMRE, a marketing agency with a focus on health care. Working in teams, participants used a preprinted template to imagine introducing a treatment device to a newly diagnosed diabetes patient. The template is similar to those used for storyboards, but it has multiple tiers of content, showing what a person is doing and feeling. Preprinted worksheets are useful for organizing this exercise.

MULTIFACETED JOURNEYS A journey map can be linear (depicting a single path) or nonlinear (branching off at various decision points). A map could diagram the stages of a patient's care from intake to discharge from a hospital unit, or it could list the steps involved in moving a patient from the emergency department to the ICU.

Journey maps are used extensively by designers planning complex digital products, such as an app or electronic system for managing health data. A complex journey map might have dozens of steps that require multiple pages or a roll of paper to display. Journey maps often narrate the emotional as well as the technical or transactional aspects of a user's experience.

Journey maps often chart the experience of multiple users. The timeline shown on the opposite page depicts stressful events that commonly occur during a primary care office visit. (User experience designers call areas of negative friction "pain points.") Locating pain points is an important step in designing better experiences. The top layer of the journey map shows the experience of the physician, while the bottom layer focuses on the patient. Physical actions, such as reviewing the patient's charts or meeting the patient, are paired with thoughts and uncertainties. Like a story with a beginning, a middle, and an end, the full map has three parts: intake and nurse assessment, medical encounter, and post-medical encounter.

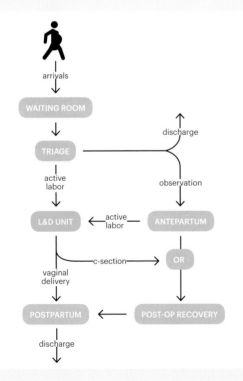

LABOR AND DELIVERY FLOW (left) This diagram shows different paths taken by patients entering the labor and delivery unit at a hospital. In a typical unit, all patients come through the waiting room and triage; then their paths diverge, depending on their clinical condition and care needs. This process map was created as part of a study conducted by Ariadne Labs, a health system innovation center, and MASS Design Group, a nonprofit architecture firm, looking at how the physical design of a hospital labor and delivery unit could lead to higher rates of cesarean deliveries.

MEDICAL ENOUNTER JOURNEY MAP

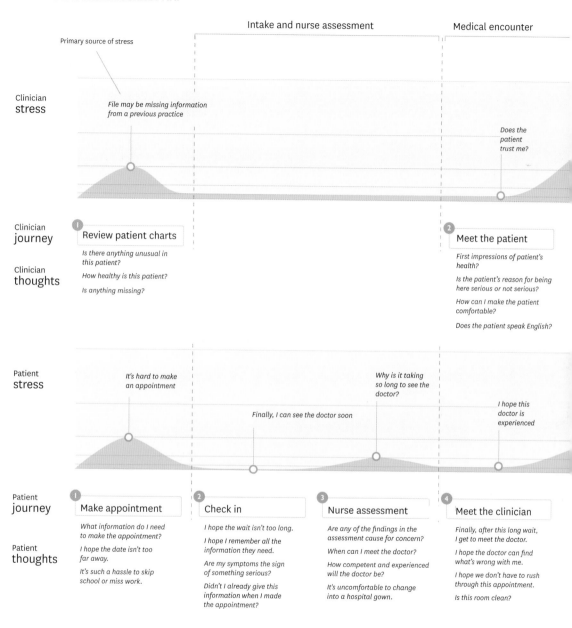

Intake and nurse assessment

Medical encounter

Primary source of stress

Clinician stress

File may be missing information from a previous practice

Does the patient trust me?

Clinician journey

1 Review patient charts

2 Meet the patient

Clinician thoughts

Is there anything unusual in this patient?

How healthy is this patient?

Is anything missing?

First impressions of patient's health?

Is the patient's reason for being here serious or not serious?

How can I make the patient comfortable?

Does the patient speak English?

Patient stress

It's hard to make an appointment

Finally, I can see the doctor soon

Why is it taking so long to see the doctor?

I hope this doctor is experienced

Patient journey

1 Make appointment

2 Check in

3 Nurse assessment

4 Meet the clinician

Patient thoughts

What information do I need to make the appointment?

I hope the date isn't too far away.

It's such a hassle to skip school or miss work.

I hope the wait isn't too long.

I hope I remember all the information they need.

Are my symptoms the sign of something serious?

Didn't I already give this information when I made the appointment?

Are any of the findings in the assessment cause for concern?

When can I meet the doctor?

How competent and experienced will the doctor be?

It's uncomfortable to change into a hospital gown.

Finally, after this long wait, I get to meet the doctor.

I hope the doctor can find what's wrong with me.

I hope we don't have to rush through this appointment.

Is this room clean?

DOUBLE-DECKER STORY (detail) The actions and thoughts of the clinician occupy the top layer, while the patient's experience unfolds on the bottom layer. Design: GoInvo

Project Board

A project board is a large vertical display that documents a team's work in progress. The board captures insights and anticipated results using words and images. The physical act of writing, sketching, and diagramming connections helps the team focus on details while maintaining a view of the big picture.

　　Why create a project visualization board? After engaging in an initial frenzy of free-flowing brainstorming and inquiry, the team needs to organize and scrutinize concepts. Project boards help design teams collect, visualize, and communicate their thinking. The flexible, inexpensive format encourages open collaboration.

　　Interesting ideas—whether in our heads or spoken aloud—are easily lost or forgotten. That's why it's important to document them. When we visualize our own ideas and those of others, we begin to open dialogue. We invite others to reflect, give feedback, and refine our work. Project boards help teams collaborate. They discourage individuals from huddling around their personal laptops writing notes or checking emails.

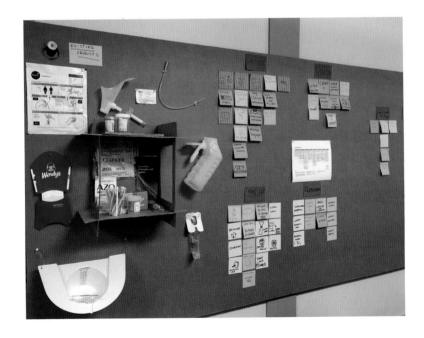

Creating a project board

1. SELECT A SURFACE

A 4×8–foot sheet of corrugated cardboard or foam core is lightweight and low cost. Material that is 1/2 inch thick works best. Use tape, thumbtacks, or drafting dots so that you can move content around and reuse the board for other projects.

2. POPULATE YOUR BOARD

Include the following elements:
—*Project title*
—*Project goals and background*
—*To-do list*
—*Charts, graphs, diagrams*
—*Journey maps*
—*Scientific articles, abstracts*
—*Photographs and sketches*
—*Artifacts and prototypes*
—*Examples or existing solutions*

3. CREATE A STRUCTURE

Allow space for capturing brainstorm sessions and compiling sticky notes, sketches, and diagrams. Look for patterns and relationships. Don't be afraid to change the layout of your board. Think of it as an organic, interactive document that evolves with your project.

4. ARCHIVE YOUR INSIGHTS

The board will quickly become overcrowded with artifacts and sketches. Declutter the project board by removing irrelevant material. Preserve your insights and ideas by capturing the content with a camera before removing it. Print these photos and place them on a corner of your board. They will act as your board's "hard drive" and can be easily referenced throughout the project.

COLLAGE OF IDEAS These project boards combine diverse materials, including artifacts and prototypes. Layers of physical data are easier to manipulate than drawings or sketches applied directly to the board. Keep the process loose and approachable, using simple materials. Posting ideas on a board helps us to map out the direction of a project. Visualize the core components of the design process (observe, imagine, and make). There is no one right way to create a project board. Each one has its own style and approach.

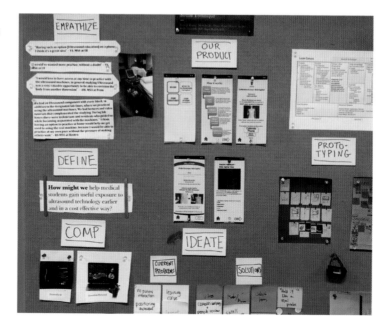

Data Visualization

Information graphics tell stories about data. Line graphs and bar charts represent numbers visually, helping us to compare them quickly and intuitively. Maps, diagrams, and illustrations make verbal explanations more understandable—like pictures in a cookbook or drawings in an anatomy textbook. Medical journals and conference presentations are packed with scattergrams, histograms, pie charts, and box plots. There are dozens of ways to visualize any single data set; a few basic approaches are explored here. When designed well, visualizations make data more meaningful.

Indeed, data graphics are part of the history of medical innovation. Florence Nightingale prevented thousands of soldier deaths during the Crimean War in the 1850s. She created a famous diagram showing that more British soldiers were dying in hospitals from unsanitary conditions and preventable infections (blue areas) than from battlefield injuries (pink areas). Nightingale's research and activism led to improved hygiene policies, first in war hospitals and then in general-use hospital wards. She is considered the founder of both modern nursing and the field of applied statistics.

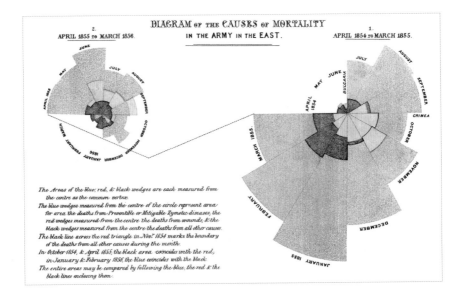

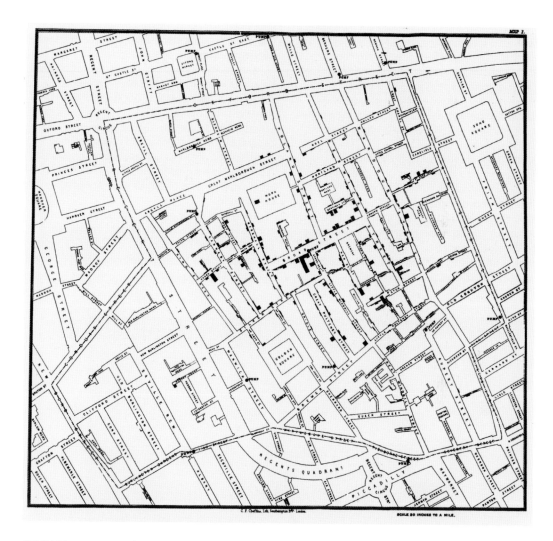

POLAR AREA DIAGRAM (opposite) Florence Nightingale's visualization of war casualities (1858) is an example of a polar area diagram, also called a rose diagram. This type of graph, which Nightingale invented, divides a circle into wedges with equal angles but different lengths. (In contrast, a pie chart slices a circle into wedges with different angles but equal lengths.) Polar area diagrams are used to plot changes taking place in a cycle. Nightingale's diagram shows the number of deaths each month over the course of a year.

DOT DENSITY MAP (above) The English physician John Snow helped found the field of epidemiology. His dot density map (1854) shows multiple cases of cholera clustered around a particular water pump in London. The map, which was drawn by Charles Cheffins, demonstrated that the disease was carried through contaminated water rather than via bad air.

READ MORE Edward Tufte, *The Visual Display of Quantitative Information*, 2nd ed. (New Haven: Graphics Press, 2001).

BAR CHARTS can be arranged in vertical or horizontal formats, depending on your layout and the quantity of data. (Horizontal bars work well for displaying a long list of categories on a vertical page.) Bar charts are used to compare data from different categories, such as *hospital/home/nursing home*. A stacked bar chart breaks down numbers within each category (such as *heart disease/cancer/diabetes*), creating a richer concentration of detail within a single chart.

LINE GRAPHS (also called line charts) are created by plotting numbers on a grid that is ordered by an x/y axis. The dots are connected to create a line. Line graphs typically show values changing over time, such as the rise and fall of a publicly traded stock. Heart monitors use line graphs to display a patient's vital signs. Data visualizations are created with standard tools such as PowerPoint, Excel, and Adobe Illustrator.

MAPS AND DIAGRAMS Spatial representations of data include geographical maps, architectural floor plans, and drawings of human anatomy. Cycle diagrams, network visualizations, and mind maps depict processes or relationships.

Geographical maps can be overlaid with other data. A flow map shows the spatial movement of people or resources; the thickness of the line represents the number. A heat map uses color to represent a variable; the map is segmented into geographic parcels such as zip codes or voting districts. In a dot density map, objects or events (such as cholera deaths or traffic accidents) are plotted geographically to illustrate spatial distribution.

These and other modes of information design can be applied to countless areas of design for health care, from studying the use of space in an emergency department to documenting the health disparities in a city.

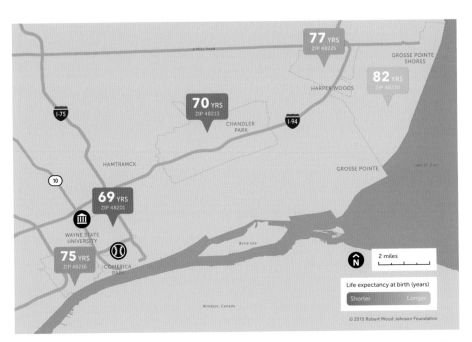

ZIP CODE GAP In many parts of the U.S., one's home address (captured by a postal zip code) is a predictor of life expectancy. Social determinants such as air quality and access to health care, education, and employment create shocking disparities in average life spans. Virginia Commonwealth University, Center on Society and Health, © Robert Wood Johnson Foundation

Basic charts, maps, and diagrams

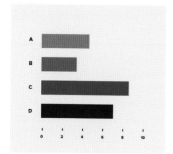

HORIZONTAL BAR CHART

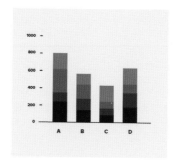

STACKED BAR CHART

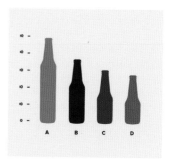

PICTORIAL BAR CHART

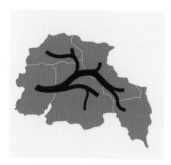

FLOW MAP

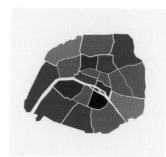

HEAT MAP

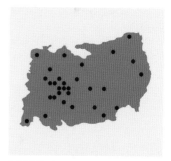

DOT DENSITY MAP

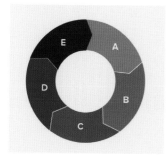

CYCLE DIGRAM

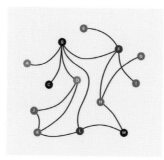

NETWORK VISUALIZATION

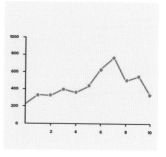

LINE GRAPH

MANY WAYS TO VISUALIZE DATA The Data Viz Project is a comprehensive archive of data visualizations, designed to help you find the right visualization and get inspired to do it. Design: Ferdio, an infographic and data visualization agency → www.datavizproject.com

VISUALIZING NUMBERS Presenting numbers as graphic points, lines, or shapes can make the relationships between quantities more concrete to a viewer. When a chart translates numbers into bars of different heights, we can quickly compare the data without having to read each number. A graph plotting a variable over time allows us to seen an overall pattern—from declining stock values to an irregular heartbeat.

An occupancy study conducted by architecture firm KieranTimberlake with the Health Design Lab at Thomas Jefferson University uses dots to represent human beings. Here, each dot indicates the location of a person in the emergency department during a particular time of day. The color of the dots matches the color on the bar charts, allowing a viewer to quickly see the times of day when the facility was more or less crowded. Again, visual information revals new insights. The data suggest that physicians were spending too much time at computer terminals at the expense of spending time with people. Potential solutions include placing stations inside patient rooms or increasing the use of notetakers (scribes) to record what is happening while the doctor focuses on delivering care.

Maggie Breslin, director of The Patient Revolution, often uses data visualization to help people consider how clinical evidence might be relevant to their lived experience. The digital tool highlighted here (opposite) supports a discussion between a woman and her clinician about whether to pursue breast cancer screening, particularly in the 40–49 age range, where guidelines have shifted and shared decision-making is recommended. The tool aims to create a space for them to talk about possible benefits, which include using early detection to avoid death, and to preclude harms such as false positives and overdiagnosis.

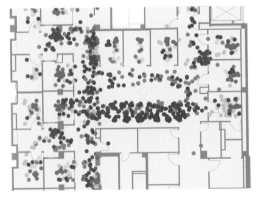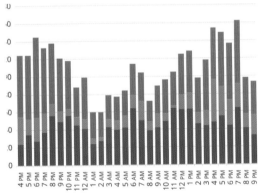

OCCUPANCY STUDY (detail) The dots represent doctors, nurses, patients, staff, and family/friends. Their locations were recorded at different hours of the day. See more: Method | Occupancy Study and Spatial Mapping. Design: KieranTimberlake

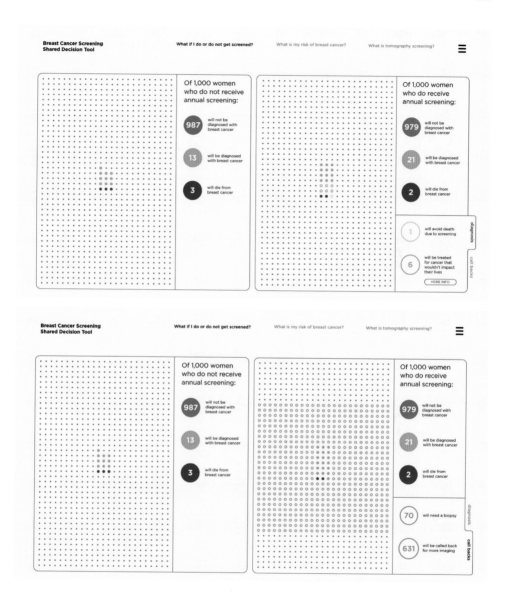

BREAST CANCER SCREENING Design: Maggie Breslin, The Patient Revolution; Leslie Ruckman. The Patient Revolution is a nonprofit organization working to develop tools, programs, and resources that help patients, caregivers, communities, and clinicians work toward health care that is careful and kind. Find out more at patientrevolution.org

VISUAL ABSTRACTS Researchers who use images and symbols to supplement their data can disseminate their scientific findings to a wider audience. Dr. Andrew Ibrahim, creator of the visual abstract, has shown how a graphical summary of a research article allows readers to understand its major findings more quickly and facilitates greater discussion. Like a trailer to a movie, a visual abstract provides a foretaste of a scientific study with simple, eye-catching visuals that make data easier to digest. Scientific evidence supports the use of visuals to rapidly and clearly communicate research findings. On average, a human requires six seconds to read twenty words but needs only a quarter of a second to extract meaning from a visual symbol. When compared with a standard text-based abstract, the articles represented by a visual abstract are shared eight times more often on social media. Leading journals and institutions, from the *New England Journal of Medicine* to the Centers for Disease Control and Prevention, have adopted this visual approach as a strategy for disseminating scientific research on social media networks and broadening the reach of knowledge.

Anatomy of a visual abstract

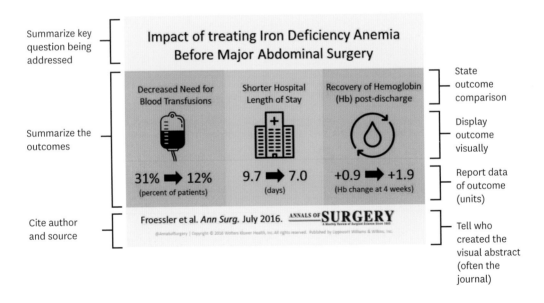

Summarize key question being addressed

Summarize the outcomes

Cite author and source

State outcome comparison

Display outcome visually

Report data of outcome (units)

Tell who created the visual abstract (often the journal)

DO IT YOURSELF You don't need to be a graphic designer to communicate visually! Learn how to create your own visual abstract → www.surgeryredesign.com/resources/

Text-based abstract vs. visual abstract

Prehospital Plasma during Air Medical Transport in Trauma Patients at Risk for Hemorrhagic Shock

J.L. Sperry, F.X. Guyette, J.B. Brown, M.H. Yazer, D.J. Triulzi, B.J. Early-Young, P.W. Adams, B.J. Daley, R.S. Miller, B.G. Harbrecht, J.A. Claridge, H.A. Phelan, W.R. Witham, A.T. Putnam, T.M. Duane, L.H. Alarcon, C.W. Callaway, B.S. Zuckerbraun, M.D. Neal, M.R. Rosengart, R.M. Forsythe, T.R. Billiar, D.M. Yealy, A.B. Peitzman, and M.S. Zenati, for the PAMPer Study Group*

ABSTRACT

BACKGROUND

After a person has been injured, prehospital administration of plasma in addition to the initiation of standard resuscitation procedures in the prehospital environment may reduce the risk of downstream complications from hemorrhage and shock. Data from large clinical trials are lacking to show either the efficacy or the risks associated with plasma transfusion in the prehospital setting.

METHODS

To determine the efficacy and safety of prehospital administration of thawed plasma in injured patients who are at risk for hemorrhagic shock, we conducted a pragmatic, multicenter, cluster-randomized, phase 3 superiority trial that compared the administration of thawed plasma with standard-care resuscitation during air medical transport. The primary outcome was mortality at 30 days.

RESULTS

A total of 501 patients were evaluated: 230 patients received plasma (plasma group) and 271 received standard-care resuscitation (standard-care group). Mortality at 30 days was significantly lower in the plasma group than in the standard-care group (23.2% vs. 33.0%; difference, −9.8 percentage points; 95% confidence interval, −18.6 to −1.0%; P=0.03). A similar treatment effect was observed across nine prespecified subgroups (heterogeneity chi-square test, 12.21; P=0.79). Kaplan–Meier curves showed an early separation of the two treatment groups that began 3 hours after randomization and persisted until 30 days

The authors' full names, academic degrees, and affiliations are listed in the Appendix. Address reprint requests to Dr. Sperry at the University of Pittsburgh, Department of Surgery and Critical Care Medicine, 200 Lothrop St., Pittsburgh, PA, 15213, or at sperryjl@upmc.edu.

*A complete list of the members of the PAMPer Study Group is provided in the Supplementary Appendix, available at NEJM.org.

Drs. Sperry and Guyette contributed equally to this article.

N Engl J Med 2018;379:315-26.
DOI: 10.1056/NEJMoa1802345
Copyright © 2018 Massachusetts Medical Society.

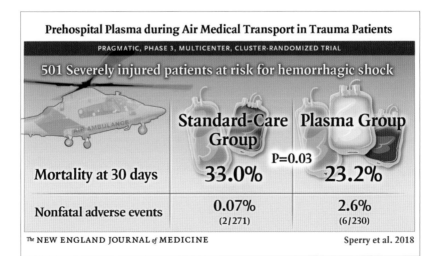

Occupancy Survey

Hospitals collect large amounts of patient data, including information like length of stay and wait times, but they rarely capture data about people's movement and behavior in the hospital. It might seem abstract to map and measure how people move around in buildings, but how can a designer, physician, or administrator make informed decisions about health care environments without having a sense of how people use them?

You can create an occupancy survey and collect data on the daily behavior of people, including their social interactions and their use of rooms, furniture, or equipment. Occupancy surveys empower building owners, students, and staff to conduct research on their own space and ask questions tailored to the challenges posed by a space. These studies can be used by health care providers to identify areas for improvement, or to support targeted interventions, such as the addition of a waiting area, before and after the implementation (see Method | Mapping the Hospital Environment).

Occupancy surveys differ from other types of questionnaire because they are spatially and temporally explicit. This means that they collect data on where people are in a space, when they are there, and what they are doing. They can be designed to study how people flow through a single room, such as a waiting room, or an entire division, such as the hospital's emergency department, over the course of a day, month, or year. An occupancy survey can also be tuned to the particular period of time relevant to a user, like a nurse's shift or a patient's full stay. Occupancy surveys can be paired with measurements of environmental factors such as sound, temperature, and lighting levels, or they can be used to create stories or maps of user experiences.

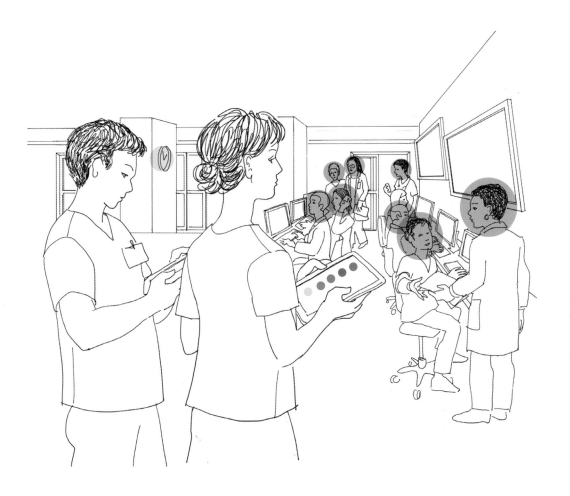

COLLECTING DATA To create a post occupancy study
(POE) of the ED at Thomas Jefferson University Hospital,
architectural researchers from KieranTimberlake and the
Health Design Lab distributed tablets to medical interns;
the tablets were loaded with a floor plan and a GIS-powered
survey application (geographic information system). The
interns collected data on the movement of nurses, doctors,
and patients, noting behaviors such as conversations,
breaks, dedicated tasks, and phone calls. They also
collected data on environmental conditions such as light,
sound, and temperature. The data was georeferenced and
time-stamped, meaning it was primed for exploration that
uses spatial mapping techniques.

SCOPE Generally, the scope of an occupancy survey is based on your goals for the data collection. Although some occupancy surveys aim to understand patterns of behavior over long periods or in typical conditions, you can also learn a lot about how people use space by observing them for shorter periods. Think about what you are trying to learn. What kind of findings would you like to report? Studies that seek to make general claims about patterns of use—for example by quantifying how many people flow through a waiting room over the course of the day, or how long a patient typically spends talking to a health care provider— require large sample sizes since there is no "average" patient or "typical" day in a hospital. For example, if you are trying to understand how much time an average patient spends speaking with a health care provider, you might need to collect data on dozens or hundreds of patients, since all will have their own experiences based on the severity of their symptoms, the busyness of the emergency department, personal communication styles, time of day, or any number of other factors.

Conversely, it can be difficult to make generalizations based on a small sample size. Sometimes the desire to generalize also leads us to discount unusual circumstances or makes us indifferent to non-normative experiences. Health care spaces have an obligation to serve all people, regardless of their differences or needs. Think about how your study can be open to and inclusive of these differences.

Occupancy surveys can also be useful for collecting qualitative data, such as user stories or observations about how different people use a space. A patient's experience of a hospital will be different from that of a nurse or a case manager. Try following a physician on her entire shift, or a patient as he navigates various areas of the hospital. Where do they go? Why? Whom do they encounter? How might the design of specific rooms affect how they feel? Observational studies can reveal information about a user's experiences that are different from your own. Try to see the space through their eyes.

SHARING RESULTS Finally, think about how your observations can be shared. Since occupancy surveys contain spatial data and observations about how people move through space, findings are often shown using maps and diagrams. A heat map can be used to overlay multiple survey instances, such as hourly snapshots of a space, to show areas of intensity or high traffic. Color can be used to differentiate among different individuals or groups in a space.

Maps can also be made to show the movement of a single person, or even of a piece of equipment. For example, could you show how a portable heart monitor is moved across a large emergency department over the course of a day? Are the patterns of movement predictable? Showing these maps to groups of users can help them think differently about how to manage their spaces.

Occupancy surveys can also produce quantitative results, such as a percentage of time spent in certain locations or doing certain activities. They can be used to answer a wide range of questions: How many people on average are in a waiting room, and at what times of day are these volumes the highest? How much time do doctors spend filling out charts as opposed to interacting with patients? How often do nurses wash their hands during a given shift? Where is the quietest location in the hospital?

Occupancy surveys often bring together quantitative and qualitative findings using a range of visualization methods. For example, to better understand how nurses care for patients, a researcher might begin by asking nurses about their work and collecting impressions of how they spend their time and what changes they might suggest for their work environment. The researcher might then shadow several nurses, noting where they go and what they do, and using the questionnaires to help focus the spatial survey. Finally, after analyzing the data, researchers might present their findings back to that group of nurses, showing them summary figures using graphs or pie charts alongside spatial maps or diagrams of their actual movement.

Planning an occupancy survey

Get permission to conduct your study.

Gather surveyors who will be collecting data.

Brainstorm research questions. What are you hoping to learn? Are your questions quantitative or qualitative? How can you make the findings spatial?

Set a survey scope. Which spaces do you want to map? For how long? Whose movement do you want to track? How much time do you have for the study?

Create a floor plan of the spaces you want to study.

Create categories of occupants (doctors, nurses, patients, family), activities (walking, talking to a patient, charting, waiting, doing a procedure), and spaces (waiting rooms, hallways, patient rooms). These categories will help you organize your findings after the survey.

Create a survey form. This will help surveyors make observations quickly and easily using defined categories. The form should also note time and locations. Use a clear floor plan or other spatial representation as a mapping background. Survey forms can be paper based or tablet based.

Test out notational strategies for drawing movement. Try using a dashed line or other symbols to represent movement or activities.

Test the survey for a short period and collect notes for improving it. Iterate!

Consider creating or using a digital platform; this can make translating large data sets much easier.

RETHINKING THE EXAM ROOM Of nearly a billion physician office visits per year in the U.S., over 50% involve primary care. The traditional exam room contains a stool, a desk, and a raised examination table covered with paper. This setup hasn't changed since the 1950s, although health care has changed significantly. One of the biggest shifts involves placing a computer in the room, owing to the adoption of electronic health records.

Medical students worked with the Health Design Lab at Thomas Jefferson University to redesign the primary care exam room. The team performed direct observations in a busy academic primary care clinic with over 80,000 visits per year. The clinic, located on the third floor of a historic building in Philadelphia, serves a diverse population ranging from people with unstable housing to executives employed in nearby offices. Students recorded how family practice doctors, trainees, nurses, medical assistants, and patients occupied the exam room. Not wanting to present

their findings in bullet points in a PowerPoint slide deck, the team sought to display their findings visually. The core design challenge was as much about changing behaviors and expectations as about changing physical spaces.

Through observational research, the team diagrammed social interactions during the doctor-patient visit. The location of the computer made it impossible for physicians to input information in the EHR (electronic health record) without literally turning their backs on patients. Furthermore, doctors could not maintain level eye contact while looking up at a person perched on a high exam table. The placement of diagnostic tools forced the physician to walk back and forth and around the exam table multiple times while performing the physical examination. Although changing the room layout may not lead to dramatic gains in efficiency, an optimized exam room could give physicians more time and better relationships with patients within their crammed fifteen-minute time slots.

Typical exam room

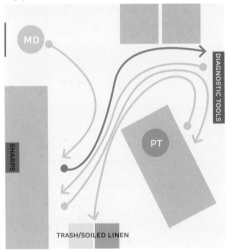

TANGLED WORKFLOW Teams documented the workflow of occupants (MD=doctor, PT=patient). Time and energy are wasted walking around the room.

Redesigned exam room

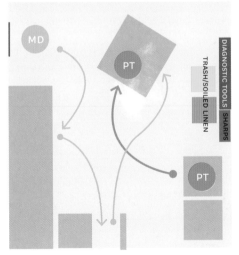

SIMPLE WORKFLOW Moving the location of a sharps container or diagnostic equipment to the opposite wall can optimize the physical layout. Diagrams redrawn based on team research; diagrams are not to scale.

Working in a poorly designed primary care exam room, a physician must turn her back to her patient in order to type notes in the EHR.

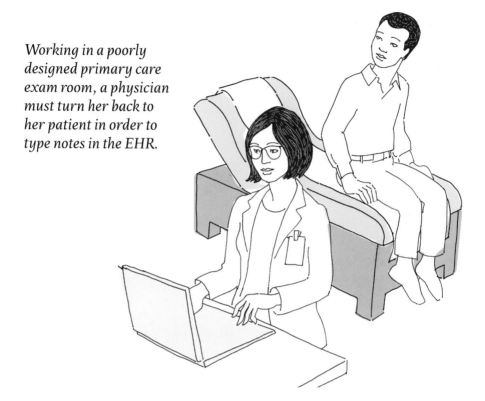

Design proposal

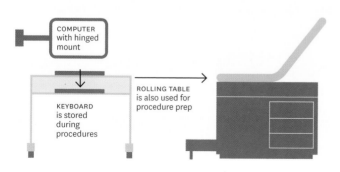

COMPUTER with hinged mount

KEYBOARD is stored during procedures

ROLLING TABLE is also used for procedure prep

Simple upgrades

Most medical practices lack big budgets to construct brand-new exam rooms. The design team at Thomas Jefferson University offered low-cost options.

Install the computer screen on a wall mount to allow face-to-face communication.

Place an extra chair in the room so that the interview can be conducted at eye level.

Reposition the otoscope/ophthalmoscope wall unit and trash can to minimize the physician's movement during the encounter.

Spatial Data Mapping

Spatial data maps use points, lines, color, shades, or hatches overlaid on an architectural floor plan to reveal how a space is used. For instance, you might be interested in mapping a snapshot of where patients and clinicians are located over a set period, such as 12, 24, or 48 hours. Or you might be interested in mapping the daily interactions between nurses and patients, or between patients and doctors. Tagged data can be assembled into spatial maps, both static and animated, using GIS or a graphics software package. Spatial maps paired with bar graphs, line graphs, or pie charts can deepen the interpretation of the data.

You can map the daily interactions between people and the hospital environment using a floor plan and data generated through occupancy surveys and environmental monitoring. Data can be collected using paper-based or tablet-based occupant survey methods. (See Method | Occupancy Survey.) Data is tagged on architectural floor plans with essential information, such as where the data is collected from, when it is collected, and what type it is.

Architectural floor plans are the base layer for spatial maps. They provide a complete layout of the area being studied, and they show adjacencies between rooms, corridors, and zones. Before collecting data, familiarize yourself with architectural floor plans and with the symbols used to represent doors, windows, and walls. Locate corridors, paths of travel, and various rooms types, such as exam, waiting, MRI, or equipment rooms. Try to layer into your floor plan information—for example about furniture and equipment—that might be relevant to the scope of your study. A basic understanding of architectural graphics will inform your approach to mapping the hospital environment. (Guides and tutorials are available online.)

After planning, designing, and implementing an occupant survey, you will have an abundant data set to play with and parse in a myriad of ways. Convene a workshop to review the data set, brainstorm study questions, and test different ways to visualize data with maps. Don't limit yourself to one question. An open mindset will allow you to examine other relationships, test alternate theories, or tell new stories.

How does occupancy in the ED change over time?

In a post occupancy study (POE) conducted at Thomas Jefferson University Hospital, the research team implemented an occupancy survey to explore how space is used in the ED. Using a snapshot approach to collecting data, medical interns mapped the location of occupants every hour over a 48-hour period. They color-coded the data to distinguish among clinicians, patients, staff, and family and friends.

The final map is paired with a bar chart showing the hourly fluctuation of the ED's population. During the study period, the number of individuals peaked early in the evening, having steadily doubled over a 14-hour period. By mapping this trend, hospital staff gained a more holistic understanding of the ED, confirmed areas of congestion, and identified opportunities for increased efficiency. The study revealed an area of high population density and congestion around the patient waiting area, adjacent nurses' station, and hallway. By visualizing their experience, staff could provide evidence to hospital administrators about how patients and clinicians competed for specific spaces on a daily basis in the ED. The ED staff reimagined the placement of the waiting room to reduce congestion and patient wait times. The study further demonstrated the potential for spatial mapping to supplement routine metrics, such as wait time and length of stay, which are statistics reported by the hospital staff regularly.

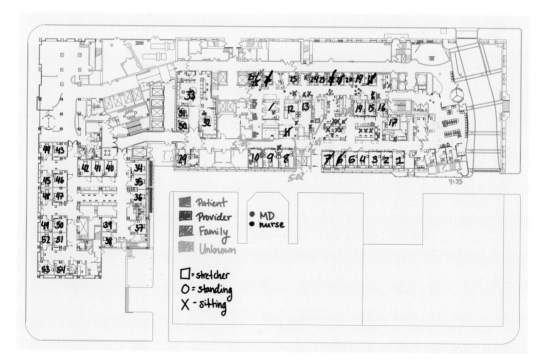

EARLY PROTOTYPES show the location of occupants in the ED. The numbers refer to patient rooms. The team used this instrument to assess whether the research interns were able to capture data answering these questions: "Who is in the ED?" "Where are they?" and "What are they doing?" Early paper prototypes like this one led to the creation of the final digital workflow, which uses geographic information systems (GIS) mapping software.

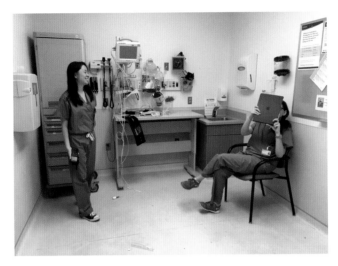

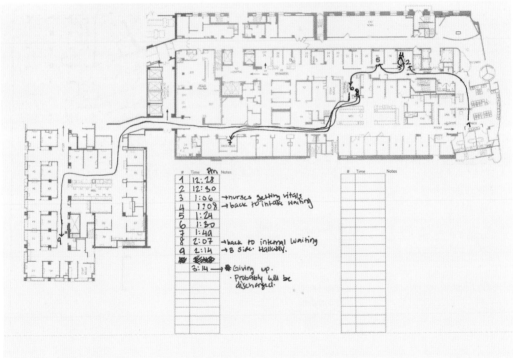

#	Time **pm**	Notes
1	12:28	
2	12:50	
3	1:06	→ nurses getting vitals
4	1:08	→ back to intake waiting
5	1:24	
6	1:30	
7	1:40	
8	2:07	→ back to internal waiting
9	2:14	→ B side hallway.
✖	✖✖✖	→ ✖ Giving up. · Probably will be discharged.
	3:14	

#	Time	Notes

RESEARCH PROCESS Researchers record light levels (top). The path of an individual is recorded by hand (bottom).

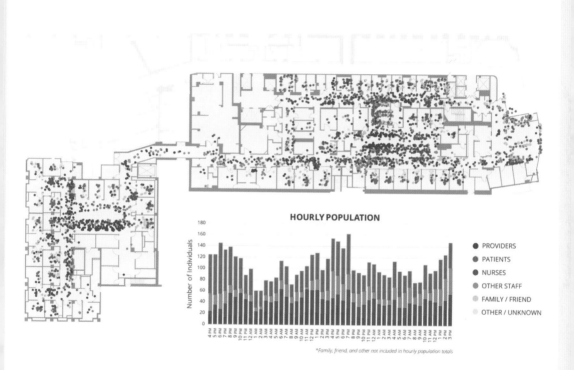

HOURLY POPULATION

Number of Individuals

- PROVIDERS
- PATIENTS
- NURSES
- OTHER STAFF
- FAMILY / FRIEND
- OTHER / UNKNOWN

*Family, friend, and other not included in hourly population totals

HOW SPACE IS USED IN THE EMERGENCY DEPARTMENT Design: KieranTimberlake

How do environmental conditions affect patient experience?

To answer this question, the design team used a shadow approach—they tracked individual patients through the ED. This method helped them understand a patient's experience over time. They used environmental sensors to measure temperature, humidity, and light and sound levels. Each person's path is accompanied by a graph of the variation in environmental conditions per space type over time.

Because people often have treatment-specific environmental requirements, variation in environmental conditions from place to place in the ED is not inherently problematic. The team understood, for example, that trauma patients

benefit from quiet environments during healing. The mapping exercise revealed spaces in the ED that were quieter or warmer than others, suggesting potential design improvements for better patient placement.

The map below reveals that a particular person interacted with various areas of the ED, interacted with several clinicians, made phone calls, watched TV, and used the restroom. The companion graph suggests that from the intake area to the patient room, this individual encountered some unevenness in ambient temperatures, especially during the first third of their experience in the ED.

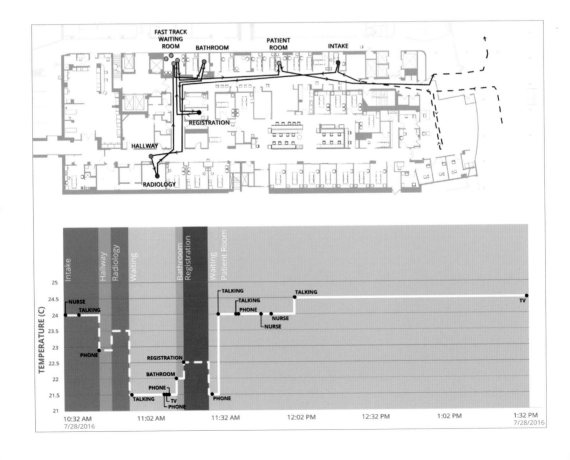

How is communication affected by different spatial arrangements?

Empowered by the results of the survey workflow and spatial mapping technique, the team initiated an additional study to target a unique spatial feature of the ED. The department is divided into two wings: the A side and B side. Therefore, the ED provided an ideal backdrop for understanding how different spatial layouts can affect communication.

The A side's centralized layout concentrates a cluster of nurses and doctors in a workstation surrounded by patient rooms, whereas the B side's decentralized layout and individual nurse stations distances the nurses from other hospital staff in situating them closer to patient rooms. Many nurses and doctors voiced strong opinions about which layout they preferred and how it affected their movement and their communication with team members. Perhaps counterintuitively, the research team's mapping paired with statistical analysis revealed that on average, the B-side's decentralized layout led to increased communication and contact time between doctors and nurses despite the greater distance between their workstations. Although this comparative study focused on existing spatial layouts in the ED, a similar method could be used to study the effects of design interventions before and after renovations.

Mapping the hospital environment allows clinicians to gain a deeper understanding of the variables that affect movement and experiences in different parts of a facility. Mapping techniques can be used to better understand, for example, the composition of a nurse's team. Quantitative analysis visualized in spatial maps does not tell the full story. The process of mapping can help designers and users of complex environments, such as an ICU, unearth patterns and possibilities for fostering more comfortable, productive, and empathetic spaces for health care.

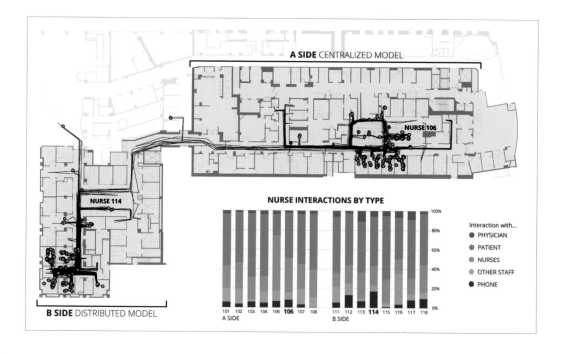

A SIDE CENTRALIZED MODEL

NURSE 106

NURSE 114

B SIDE DISTRIBUTED MODEL

NURSE INTERACTIONS BY TYPE

Interaction with...
● PHYSICIAN
● PATIENT
● NURSES
○ OTHER STAFF
● PHONE

101 102 103 104 105 **106** 107 108
A SIDE

111 112 113 **114** 115 116 117 118
B SIDE

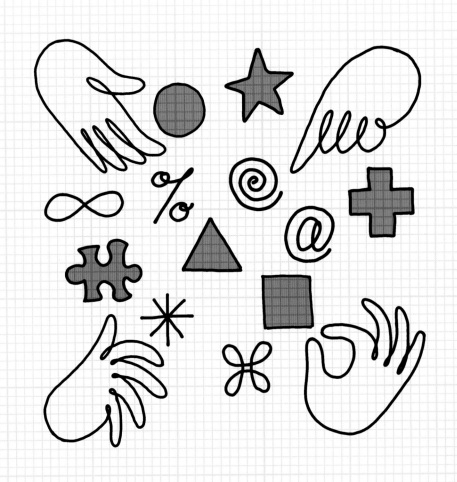

Case Studies

The following pages explore the application of health design thinking to products, services, and spaces. Although some of these endeavors are led by individuals, most represent the effort of interdisciplinary teams. These case studies are the work of clinicians, patients, designers, engineers, and entrepreneurs, carried out in the context of hospitals, medical schools, community organizations, government agencies, and health care companies. Included are fully developed commercial products along with concept proposals and research and development studies.

Prescription Drug Packaging

Deborah Adler, a graphic designer specializing in design for health care, has been improving pill bottles since 2004. That's when she launched a top-to-bottom redesign of the standard amber pill bottle as her graduate thesis project at the School of Visual Arts in New York City. Her pioneering school project became the basis of Target's ClearRx, a new approach to prescription drug packaging. Bold, simple labels are applied to a flattened, cap-down bottle, whose surface provides a bigger billboard for displaying crucial information about dosages. A color-coded ring around the bottle cap helps identify which pills belong to whom.

Adler's latest foray into pill packaging is an innovation brought to CVS Pharmacy. Adler's graphics help users understand when and how often to take a given medication and how many doses to take. This information is especially important for patients taking multiple medications, since drugs may have dangerous interactions. The label on each bottle states the patient's name in large type. A visual timeline divides the day into morning, midday, evening, and bedtime. Each quadrant has a memorable icon and color. When you line the bottles up, you can read the times of day across bottles. Similar graphics appear on an instruction sheet printed by the pharmacy.

Such tools encourage patients to take their medications safely and regularly. Many patients don't refill their recurring prescriptions—and many patients don't finish taking the first course of a prescribed medication. Noncompliance can have negative health impacts while creating needless waste (and lost revenue for the pharmacy).

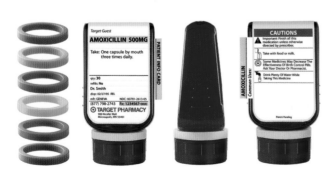

TARGET'S CLEARRX
Label system design: Deborah Adler. Industrial design: Klaus Rosburg. Photo courtesy of Target

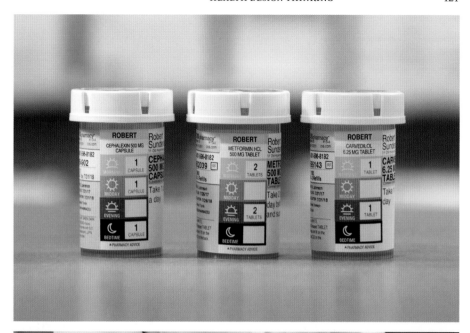

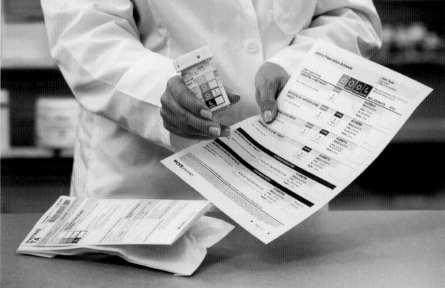

CVS PRESCRIPTION DRUG LABEL SYSTEM Deborah Adler's innovative package design, adopted by CVS Pharmacy, aims to encourage compliance and build customer loyalty with labels that are easy to read and easy to live with. When the bottles are lined up next to each other, they clearly represent the patient's daily pill regimen. Photos courtesy of CVS

READ MORE Cliff Kuang, "CVS Taps a Design Legend to Reinvent the Prescription Label. Next Stop: The Pharmacy," *Fast Company*, October 4, 2017, → fastcompany.com/90145401/cvs-taps-a-design-legend-to-reinvent-the-prescription-label-next-stop-the-pharmacy

Pharmacy Redesign

Health design thinking has the potential to transform large economic sectors. The pharmaceutical industry has the opportunity to serve the public better through improved design of services and packaging. Prescription drugs are lifesaving tools; yet according the World Health Organization, only half of patients with a chronic illness in the U.S. take a medication as prescribed. One study estimates that the lack of medication adherence causes roughly 125,000 deaths and raises U.S. health care costs by hundreds of billion dollars per year. There are many reasons for this problem, including the high cost of drugs, inadequate insurance coverage, inconvenience or a lack of privacy, and difficulty with following a drug regimen.

PillPack, a home delivery system for prescription medications, attempts to redesign the entire pharmacy experience. In seven years, PillPack went from a concept that won a health care hackathon to a full-service pharmacy company that Amazon bought for nearly $1 billion. TJ Parker, the co-founder of PillPack, is a second-generation pharmacist who took design classes alongside his pharmacy coursework during college. During the company's startup phase, Parker and his colleagues worked with designers at IDEO to refine their strategy, improve the website experience, and build their products.

Parker reinvented the antiquated process of the typical pharmacy by framing prescription drug delivery as a user experience design problem. The act of obtaining a prescription medication is inconvenient and cumbersome. You go to your local pharmacy, wait in line, and get asked within earshot of other customers if you have any questions about your prescription. Many people are hesitant to discuss drugs that reveal personal medical issues.

PillPack redesigns the entire customer journey. Although it does not address all the problems of providing medications to people, it reduces the pain points of traveling to a pharmacy, refilling prescriptions, and sorting out and scheduling multiple medications with a pill box at home.

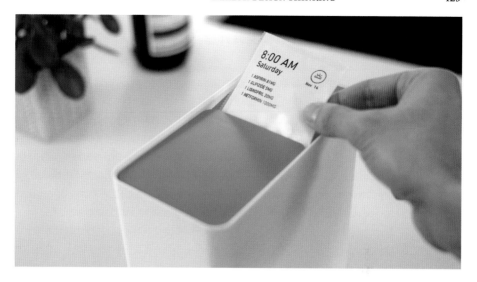

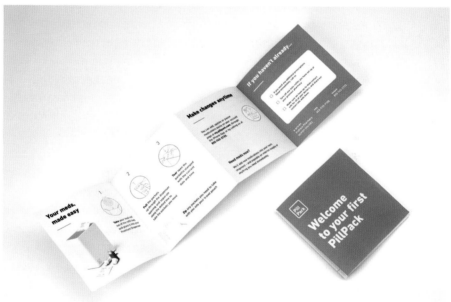

NO MORE BOTTLES A roll of presorted pills arrives every two weeks. The patient loads the roll into a dispenser box. The presorted packets have easy-to-read text showing the drug's name, the correct dosage, and the exact time and date to take it. The printed manual employs visual illustrations and instructions written in simple language. The clearly labeled, ready-to-use pack can prevent medication errors such as taking the wrong pill or missing or repeating a dose.

READ MORE Emily Dreyfuss, "The Pharmacy of the Future Is Ready For Your Bathroom Counter," *Wired*, June 15, 2017, → wired.com/story/pillpack-pharmacy-of-the-future-is-ready-for-your-bathroom/. Meera Viswanathan, PhD, *et al.*, "Interventions to Improve Adherence to Self-administered Medications for Chronic Diseases in the United States: A Systematic Review," *Annals of Internal Medicine* 157, no. 11 (2012): 785–95.

Surgical Procedure Trays

Deborah Adler's philosophy of health care is inspired by the concept of "lean manufacturing," pioneered by Toyota in Japan in the 1930s. Toyota revolutionized the car industry by shifting the emphasis from producing many identical parts for many identical products (as Henry Ford had done) to creating smaller batches of parts for smaller batches of products. This strategy resulted in a brilliant confluence of efficiency and product variety. As Adler has discussed, the Japanese term *gemba* refers to the real place where the work is done. For Toyota, the gemba is the factory floor. For a journalist, it might be the scene of a crime. For a doctor or nurse, it's the patient's bedside. For a pharmacist, it could be where drugs are made or the patient's medicine cabinet.

Adler observes that lean methods are being applied to health care, which seeks to control cost by ending waste, delivering more consistent care, creating a patient-centered experience, and reducing readmissions. For Adler, "going to the gemba" means watching and observing the many places in a hospital where health care is in production. One of these places is the central sterile supply room. This is where surgical procedure trays are kept. A unique tray of sterile tools is needed for any given procedure, from brain surgery to a total hip replacement. The material manager is responsible for supplying the correct tray to the scrub tech. If the wrong tray is delivered and opened, it gets thrown away, a waste of hundreds of dollars. There is also the risk of inadvertently exposing sensitive patients to latex.

Adler, working with the hospital supply company Medline, reorganized the storage system as well as the packaging. The new trays are still blue, but each one has a colored belly band that identifies the general type of surgery, such as eyes/nose/throat. Related trays are stored together. The new system addresses multiple aspects of health care delivery: communication, technology, and safety. Hospitals are trying to become 99% waste free, and projects like this are helping. The new trays save money by rationalizing the work of stocking and picking, and they reduce the danger, inconvenience, and expense that result from wrong choices.

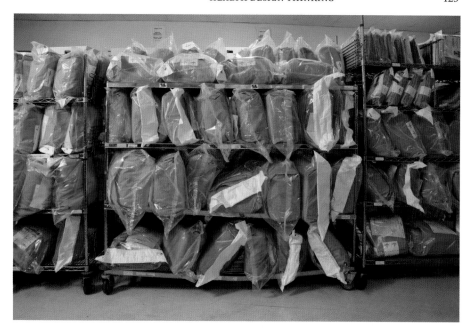

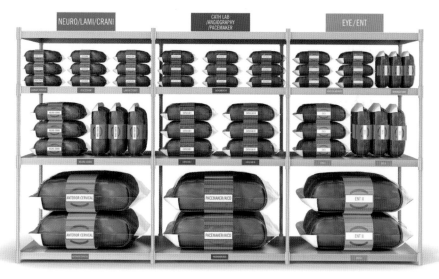

MEDLINE SURGICAL PROCEDURE TRAYS A jumble of blue bags fills the central sterile supply room (top). "It's crazy town," says designer Deborah Adler. "All the packs are big, bulky, and blue—and not Tiffany blue." In the prototype for the redesigned packaging system (bottom), tray packs are grouped and color-coded according to the type of surgery to be performed.

Foley Catheter Kit

Traditional catheter kits have a double tray setup. Most of the pieces required for the procedure are packed into the top tray, and the catheter is wound tightly in the bottom tray. The sterile trays provide a work area for the nurse, and this area is very small, making the process awkward, uncomfortable, and prone to error. The catheter has a tendency to fall off the sterile field, becoming contaminated and causing infection.

Deborah Adler designed a new package for Medline that creates a "calmer and more sterile experience." On a single-layer tray, the elements are packed in the sequence in which the nurse will use them, instead of being jammed wherever they happen to fit. The one-layer tray creates more space for the nurse to work by providing a bigger playing field. Many patients are unnecessarily catheterized so they won't have to use bedpans. This is a common source of infections. The new package includes a stop-and-check protocol to help prevent unnecessary catheter use.

The new one-layer tray worked well, but the design team observed that nurses were tossing away the patient education material included in the kit. Adler commissioned an illustrator to create a beautiful Hallmark-type card with the patient information inside. The card is special and personal, so nurses don't discard it. Patients put it on their bedside table, where it also serves to educate the family. Because of its beauty and tactility, the card was perceived as a thing of value.

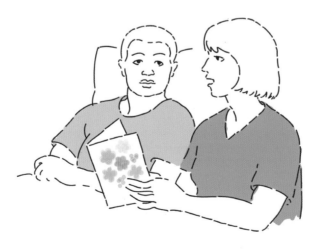

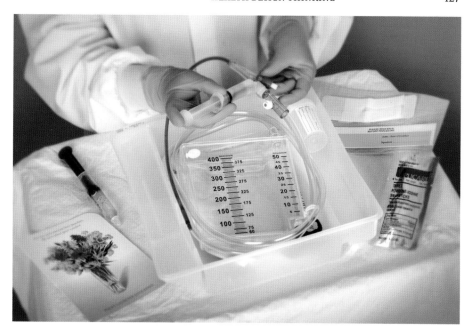

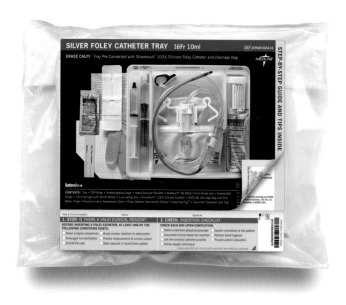

MEDLINE FOLEY CATHETER KIT The graphics on the outside of the package explain how to insert a catheter. (The instructions unfold from behind an informative photograph of the contents of the kit.)

Hospital Garments

For cancer patients receiving chemotherapy through a peripherally inserted central catheter (PICC) line, the standard of care sometimes includes a sawed-off tube sock. This bulky, frayed sock holds the port in place just above the elbow, and it has to be worn for the duration of treatment (weeks, months, or even years). Chaitenya Razdan (Care+Wear Co-Founder and CEO), who was a Wall Street investment banker at the time, learned about the tube sock problem from a friend who had recently been diagnosed with cancer. Oncologists at Johns Hopkins Hospital took interest in Razdan's idea to make a better PICC line cover. The tube sock solution is both troubling for nurses and demeaning for patients. The sock doesn't adequately hold the line in place, leading to potential infection when the line rips away.

Razdan teamed up with co-founder Susan Jones and clinicians from Hopkins to design a purpose-built PICC Line Cover. Made from ultrasoft, antimicrobial materials, the cover is sporty, comfortable, and secure. A transparent window allows the site to be monitored for infection. Care+Wear creates a wide range of patient-centered clothing. Codesigned with patients and clinicians, each piece supports the dignity and comfort of patients while optimizing the treatment process. The Care+Wear line includes shirts and hoodies for accessing ports on the chest, a functional and attractive patient gown, and a one-piece infant garment (onesie) designed for premature infants in the NICU. These and other pieces are available online and through hospitals and health systems.

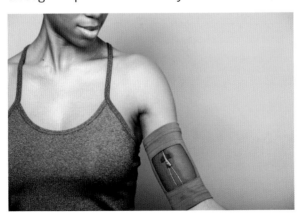

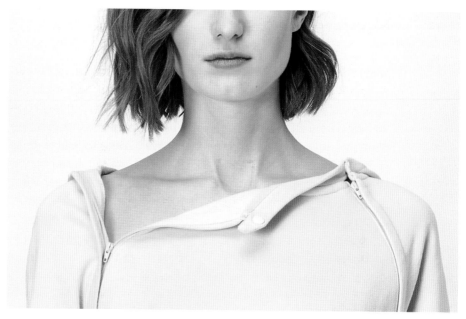

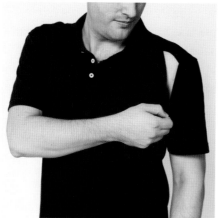

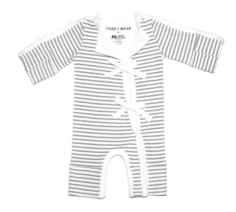

CARE+WEAR Ultra-Soft, Antimicrobial PICC Line Cover (opposite page); Oscar de la Renta Port Access Hoodie (top); Chest & Port Access Shirt (bottom left); March of Dimes NICU Preemie Onesie. Photos courtesy of Care+Wear

READ MORE Kim Olsen, "Oscar de la Renta Partners with Maryland Native to Debut Hoodies for Cancer Patients," *Washingtonian*, May 3, 2018, → www. washingtonian.com/2018/05/03/oscar-de-la-renta-partners-with-maryland-native-to-debut-hoodies-for-cancer-patients/

Hospital Hacks

Molly Bonnell and her sister were born with cystic fibrosis, a serious chronic illness requiring frequent hospitalization and ongoing medical care. As a fashion design student at Parsons School of Design in New York City, Bonnell sought to develop a new approach to hospital garments. She wondered why patients have to wear special clothing at all. The typical hospital gown is designed to make it easier for clinicians to access the patient's body while administering care. Such garments are not only impersonal and undignified—they are also uncomfortable. Bonnell believes that patient garments should be warm and comforting to the skin, and they should affirm a patient's humanity and individuality.

Called Hospital Hacks, Bonnell's experimental project includes comfortable, relaxed clothes, such as T-shirts and sweaters that have been fitted with functional openings tailored for hospital use. The clothing can also be worn outside the hospital, since people often attend to their medical needs at home, at work, and in other nonmedical settings. Bonnell has also created embroidered patches, stamps, and other supplies that invite patients to customize their own garments. How-to manuals make the process fun and engaging; they encourage patients to express pride in their medical experience as a "badge of honor."

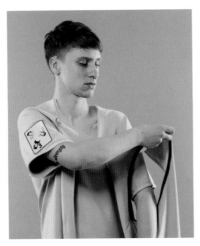 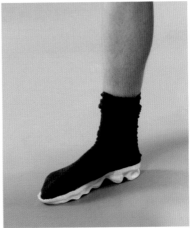

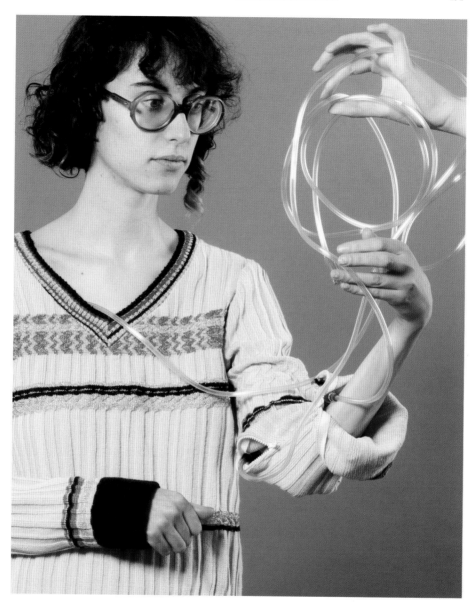

EASY ACCESS Through her research with patients and clinicians, Molly Bonnell learned that Velcro is a poor material for hospital garments because bacteria can thrive among its tiny hooks and loops. She used plastic zippers because metal is incompatible with MRI and X-ray machines. Her project includes improved hospital slippers (opposite, right) and garments whose zippers are carefully positioned for convenience and style (above). Bonnell also designed a hospital gown to be worn during procedures (opposite, left). The gown provides more coverage by wrapping around the body; it has no ties or belts. All pieces are designed with the rigors of hospital laundry in mind. Photography: Brandon Petulla

READ MORE Leanne Prain, "A Wardrobe for Wellness," *Works That Work* 10 (2017), → worksthatwork.com/10/humanising-the-hospital-experience-through-design

Wearable Diagnostics

Many medical diagnostics suffer from bad design. The equipment is bulky and cumbersome, and it typically requires a medical professional when it's used within a clinic or hospital setting. As advances in technology yield faster and smaller processors, creating portable diagnostic medical equipment has become more feasible. Design plays a critical role in ensuring that people without medical backgrounds can safely use digital health devices.

AliveCor's Kardiamobile, a device the size of a credit card, syncs with a smartphone and allows users to generate their own electrocardiograms (ECGs). The Kardia app can interpret heart tracings and detect abnormal heart rhythms such as atrial fibrillation (a known cause of stroke).

In 2018, Apple enhanced its popular Apple Watch, shifting it from fitness tracker and high-end accessory into the digital health realm by creating two new features: an ECG app and fall detection. The ECG feature allows the user to simply place a finger on the digital crown to create an ECG tracing, without the need for an external device. The ECG app detects atrial fibrillation and accelerated heart rates, and it shares data with medical professionals. The fall detection app uses the accelerometer within the watch to monitor and detect falls.

Both the AliveCor Kardiamobile and the Apple Watch carry a U.S. Food and Drug Administration Class II clearance. The ability of digital health to make health care more convenient, safe, and accessible will continue to depend upon the integration of design into the process of creating, testing, and implementing products and devices.

As doctors, patients, and health care systems embrace new technologies, from wearable diagnostics to artificial intelligence, it is critical to understand their limitations and be aware of potential downfalls, such as data breaches of personal health information. Having a beautifully designed interface for a wearable medical device does not guarantee that the device will reliably capture your health data, present the data accurately, or secure your privacy. Designers of medical products should apply the same ethical principle that physicians apply in their practice: "First, do no harm."

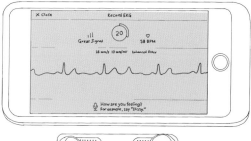

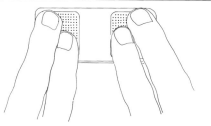

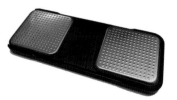

ALIVECOR KARDIAMOBILE DEVICE The user places the index and middle fingers of each hand on the pads to generate an ECG tracing on a compatible mobile phone. By 2017, the device had recorded over 20 million ECGs. AliveCor is working to develop additional capabilities for the device, including detection of prolonged QT syndrome (a heart rhythm disorder) and hyperkalemia (high potassium blood level).

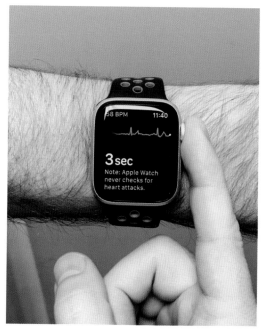

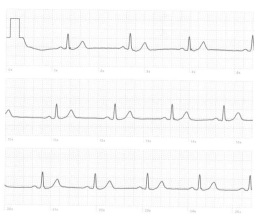

APPLE WATCH SERIES 4 The user places an index finger on the digital crown to generate an ECG tracing on the iPhone ECG App that can then be shared with a medical professional. When a sudden impact occurs, the fall detection app alerts emergency services and sends messages to the owner's emergency contacts.

iBreastExam

iBreastExam is a device created for early detection of breast cancer, for use in areas without access to mammography. In 2009, Mihir Shah, Matthew Campisi, and Bhaumik Sanghvi set out to create a low-power, low-cost, radiation-free device that could deliver results on the spot and be used safely and effectively by community health workers (CMWs) worldwide. In 2009, they co-founded UE LifeSciences, a company now operating in India, Malaysia, and the U.S. The design principle behind iBreastExam is "MLM,"or "more from less for more." The product has a simple design and a small number of components; it is usable by someone with no medical education or medical device experience.

The project got off the ground in 2012, when the team won a grant for nearly $1 million from the Pennsylvania Department of Health. The challenge was to develop a new mechanism for early detection of breast cancer among underserved populations. These populations are everywhere—from Malaysia to Mexico to New York City. Breast cancer is spreading quickly across the developing world, as more communities adopt elements of the Western lifestyle, including smoking, alcohol, sedentary behavior, processed foods, meat-based diets, and later childbirth. While breast cancer is spreading, access to early detection is not.

Shah, who teaches a course in biomedical entrepreneurship at Drexel University in Philadelphia, PA, explains that creating a medical device for the developing world is like playing chess with yourself. In order to succeed, you must satisfy multiple criteria, such as a portable power source, extreme usability, small data packets requiring minimal bandwidth, and pain-free, radiation-free treatment. The device must be able to withstand extreme dust and humidity, and, above all, it must hit a high bar in clinical efficacy. It has to work.

iBreastExam has been validated by multiple medical journals. It has been used to screen over 200,000 women in twelve countries. UE LifeSciences has gathered support from University of Pennsylvania Abramson Cancer Center, Drexel University, and GE Healthcare. Manufactured in India, the product uses culturally appropriate technologies to address global health care disparities.

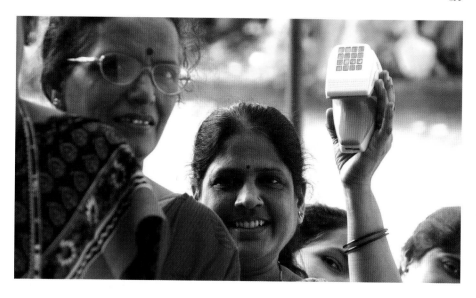

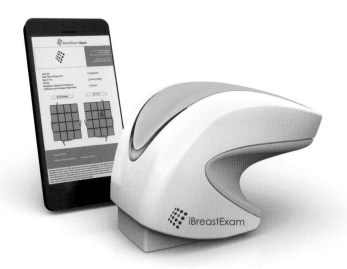

USER-FRIENDLY The physical product has no buttons except for on/off. It is battery operated and can be used by a community health worker with minimal training. Photos courtesy of UE LifeSciences

Developers: Mihir Shah, Matthew Campisi, and Bhaumik Sanghvi, UE LifeSciences. Product design: Ian White, DesignDesign. Design for manufacturability: Design Directions, India

READ MORE Robyn B. Broach, Rula Geha, Brian S. Englander, Lucy DeLaCruz, Holly Thrash, and Ari D. Brooks, "A Cost-effective Handheld Breast Scanner for Use in Low-resource Environments: A Validation Study," *World Journal of Surgical Oncology* 14 (2016), → doi.org/10.1186/s12957-016-1022-2

SOLUTIONS THAT WORK The creators of iBreastExam do not claim that their product is better than mammography. Rather, they assert that it is more suited to many developing-world contexts where the equipment is prohibitively expensive and radiologists may not be present. Such a workforce is simply not available in regions like India or China. Furthermore, cultural resistance to mammograms exists in many communities. Women don't want to submit to a painful procedure that exposes them to radiation. Finally, mammography is not very effective in populations of younger women, who have denser breast tissue than older women.

How can a breast lesion be detected? The tumor is harder than the surrounding breast tissue. In a manual exam, a trained clinician is seeking a hard, immobile structure within the breast. By the time a lesion can be felt manually, however, the disease is already advanced and will progress quickly, becoming metastatic.

iBreastExam does not use ultrasound. Why not? Because experts are required to interpret ultrasound results. In many countries, including India and Brazil, only a board-certified technician is permitted to interpret ultrasound results.

iBreastExam features a tactile sensor. Activated by physical contact with the skin, the sensor detects tissue stiffness by pressure. Using sensor technology invented at Drexel University, the device converts mechanical pressure into electrical signals, assessing the stiffness of tissue in real time.

Imagine a pillow filled with soft feathers or fluffy foam. Now, imagine searching for a small, hard ball deep inside the pillow. As you feel something stiffer, it will exert pressure in the opposite direction.

iBreastExam aims to to find tumors that are not yet large enough to be palpable to the hand, at a size between 5mm and 15mm. These are clinically relevant breast lesions—tumors that represent invasive breast cancer. iBreastExam is unable to detect microcalcification, a form of pre-cancer. Cell abnormalities at such an early stage may be better left undetected. The health care system in a developing region would be overwhelmed if every case of pre-cancer were treated, and women would be plunged into needless anxiety.

"You are not just making a product—you are designing for an entire cultural ecosystem."

MIHIR SHAH

OPERABLE, SCALABLE BREAST CANCER SCREENING IN LIMITED-RESOURCE SETTINGS

GOLD-STANDARD MODALITIES	ACCESSIBLE & AFFORDABLE	USABLE W/MINIMAL TRAINING	SCALABLE & CLOUD-CONNECTED	STANDARDIZED & OBJECTIVE
Mammography	✗	✗	✗	✔
Breast Ultrasound	✗	✗	✗	✔
Clinical Breast Exam	✔	✗	✗	✗
iBreastExam	✔	✔	✔	✔

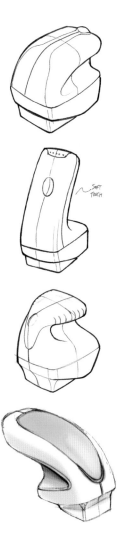

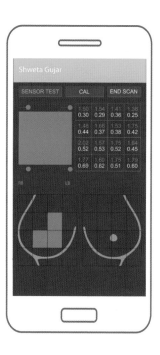

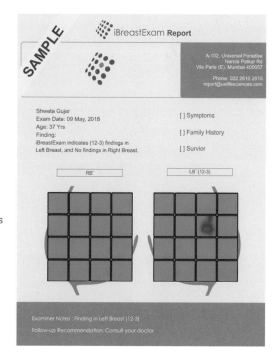

PORTABLE AND COMPACT DesignDesign, a product design firm in Kennett Square, Pennsylvania, sketched and prototyped numerous concepts for the physical device, which must house the technological components in addition to supporting comfortable and intuive use. iBreastExam connects via bluetooth to a mobile device. Data is collected on the phone, which displays an image of the breast. The technician taps an area of the breast shown on the screen and then scans that area. The phone and the mobile app act as a monitor. The app generates a PDF report that can be emailed to the patient or the doctor, for use via direct consultation or telemedicine.

Newborn Phototherapy

Design That Matters (DtM) creates context-appropriate medical devices for use in developing communities. DtM founder Timothy Prestero and his colleagues have developed human-centered design principles tailored to the needs of underresourced hospitals.

Global health experts estimate that 5–10% of all newborn mortality is due to jaundice, despite the fact that jaundice is so easy to cure simply by shining blue light on the baby's skin. The DtM design team found that existing phototherapy devices are easy to misuse, meaning that in many cases jaundice is not treated effectively. Firefly is a newborn phototherapy device designed to allow rural hospitals with limited resources and minimally trained staff to successfully treat otherwise healthy newborns for jaundice at the point of diagnosis, rather than risk transporting them to crowded central facilities. Unlike the conventional overhead phototherapy devices hospitals might receive through international donations or government purchase, Firefly provides high-intensity phototherapy that is "hard to use wrong"—in other words, the device eliminates the most common sources of product failure.

Although phototherapy is a simple treatment, it is often administered inappropriately. Most overhead devices have adjustable height settings, but when positioned incorrectly, they fail to provide the right treatment. Despite the fact that overhead phototherapy devices are intended to treat one infant at a time, clinicians in overcrowded hospitals routinely treat multiple infants in the same device at once. Then all the treated infants receive ineffective doses of phototherapy and face a higher risk of cross infection. By integrating the infant bed into the product's overall design and placing the lights at a nonadjustable, fixed distance, Firefly prevents users from providing the wrong dose of phototherapy to the patient and prevents hospitals from placing more than one infant in the device. The curved canopy discourages clinicians from resting objects on top of the light, making the product even safer to use.

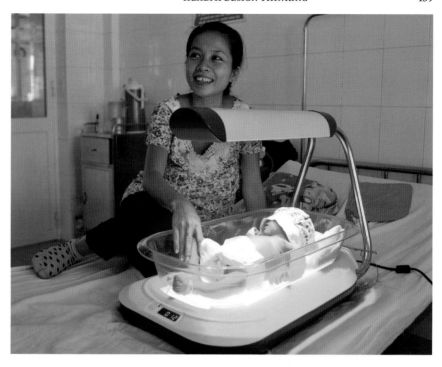

OVERHEAD PHOTOTHERAPY

FIREFLY PHOTOTHERAPY

TOP LIGHT

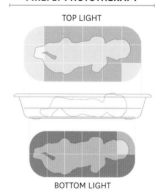

IRRADIANCE
µW/cm²/nm
00 - 10
10 - 20
20 - 30
30 - 40
40 - 50

EFFECTIVE PHOTOTHERAPY

INTENDED USE

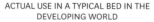

ACTUAL USE IN A TYPICAL BED IN THE
DEVELOPING WORLD

BOTTOM LIGHT

FIREFLY The design of the device makes it "hard to use wrong." The bassinet fits one infant instead of many, reducing the risk of cross infection. Because Firefly shines light from below as well as from above, it reduces treatment time by at least 40% compared with state-of-the-art single-sided LED phototherapy. Firefly's LEDs last up to 44,000 hours, and the device operates at just 30 watts— up to 70% less than other common phototherapy systems. Firefly is small, so it can be used in the mother's recovery room. Firefly promotes breastfeeding, encourages mother–child bonding, and leads to superior treatment. The rounded, seamless bassinet can be wiped clean in seconds. The outer casings have tight seams and no vents, which prevents insects, dust, and liquids from damaging the device or dimming the lights. Internal moving parts have been eliminated, including fans, which can be easily broken.

READ MORE Text adapted from → www.designthatmatters.org/firefly

Behavioral Health

Numerous individuals who seek mental health specialty care are below the clinical threshold for depression and anxiety. Many communities and health care networks lack a systematic way to offer these nonspecialty services.

Kaiser Permanente (KP), a not-for-profit health plan and a network of hospitals and medical groups operating across the United States, created Project Chamai to improve emotional health. This service aims to meet growing demand from members and employers for accessible, affordable options for emotional health and well-being. Project Chamai seeks to help prevent the worsening of symptoms and promote overall health while allowing KP to focus specialty care resources on those with more acute needs.

Project Chamai is a prevention and early intervention system for patients with mild to moderate emotional health symptoms. The ecosystem includes web- and mobile-based content (articles, videos, and podcasts); an online personal action plan (OPAP); a KP content hub; and "digital therapeutics" in the form of third-party applications and online programs. Chamai includes "digital prescription" capabilities for these resources in primary and specialty care, along with outreach to members upstream.

KP conducted interviews, observations, and chart reviews in efforts to understand the needs and experiences of members and staff. Members actively participated in defining the core values and features of the Chamai ecosystem. KP reports an encouraging level of engagement from members who have enrolled in Chamai.

KP has been applying human-centered design to health care since 2003. Design-driven innovations at KP have included making hospital-to-home transitions more patient-centered, creating better nurse shift change processes, and transforming the design of ambulatory clinics and hospitals.

PROJECT CHAMAI ECOSYSTEM

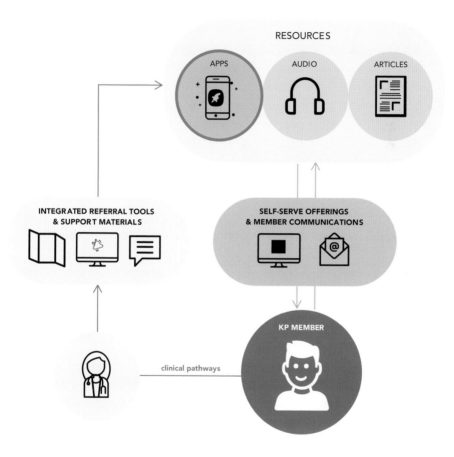

Digital Therapeutics

Health care is increasingly being delivered via digital applications rather than through brick-and-mortar facilities, so the appropriate and ethical design of mobile apps, health data software, and wireless medical devices has become crucial. The design of digital interfaces in health care affects millions of lives. Bad design in digital health—just like a doctor's poor bedside manner—can have negative effects on a patient's health. Patients who interact with a clunky or confusing digital product will disengage. The majority of people who download a health app stop using it. Clinicians and nurses also feel the repercussions of poor design. EHRs promised to revolutionize health care by increasing physician efficiency and improving patient experiences; instead, the EHR has become a major driver for physician burnout. The failed design of EHRs spawned a new industry: medical scribes. These notetakers are a workaround to the burden of documentation and clerical work created by EHRs.

Digital therapeutics is an emerging field of medicine. For patients with chronic diseases requiring behavioral modification, digital therapeutics can be as effective as prescription drugs for achieving better health outcomes. The main ingredient for digital therapeutics is the design of the software and its interface. A well-designed app or website will engage patients, remind them of their health goals, and motivate healthier behaviors.

Omada Health is one of the first companies to be recognized by the Centers for Disease Control and Prevention for delivering digital therapeutics that meet evidence-based guidelines for preventing type 2 diabetes. Founders Sean Duffy and Adrian James used design thinking principles to conceive of a digital behavioral management program to prevent the onset of type 2 diabetes, research they began while working at the design firm IDEO. Their concept met IDEO's trifecta for business innovation: desirability, feasibility, and viability. Omada Health's evidence-based methodology, results-based business model, and user-friendly experience design has helped make their platform an industry leader in digital therapeutics. People enrolled in their program have high rates of sustained engagement and statistically significant reductions in risk factors for chronic disease.

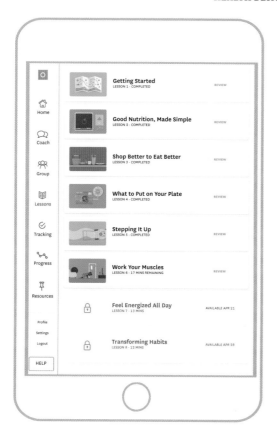

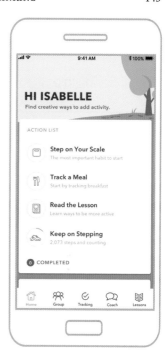

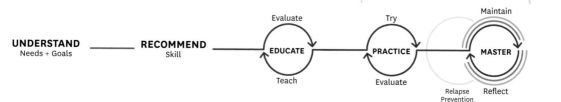

UNDERSTAND — Needs + Goals ——— RECOMMEND — Skill ——— EDUCATE (Evaluate / Teach) — PRACTICE (Try / Evaluate) — MASTER (Maintain / Reflect / Relapse Prevention)

CHANGING BEHAVIOR (top) The Omada platform includes a digital app for a tablet or phone and a wirelessly connected digital bathroom scale. The app is used to track food consumption, complete interactive lessons, communicate with a professional health coach and peer group, and receive alerts and reminders. Omada offers its service through health insurers, health systems, and employers rather than marketing directly to consumers. Omada's pricing model is based on results: the company earns fees when participants enroll in the program and meet specific goals.

(above) Omada's Product Design team created a behavior journey map based on hundreds of participant interviews. The map guides teams at Omada Health to build products, optimize processes, and help people to maintain healthier habits. Design: Product design team, Omada Health

READ MORE Stanford Byers Center for Biodesign, October 25, 2017, → biodesign.stanford.edu/content/dam/sm/biodesign/documents/case-studies/Omada-Health-Establishing-Long-Term-Business-Viability.pdf

Digital Health Record

The Chicago-based design firm Greater Good Studio used the principles and methods of health design thinking—prototyping, codesign, user testing, and storyboarding—to develop a point-of-care digital health record for community health workers in Rwanda. The Ihangane Project, a nonprofit organization promoting high-quality primary health care in rural communities, needed a better way for their community health workers to record clinical data and report that data to the Rwanda Ministry of Health. The usual method of collecting data involving handwritten measurements on paper was time-consuming and cumbersome. Earlier efforts to make this process paperless in rural health centers resulted in an electronic health record system that was complicated, required additional staff support, and added to the workload of existing staff.

The design team faced challenges: poor internet access, barriers to adoption of a new tool, and the need to make their solution compatible with the software program used by the Rwanda Ministry of Health District. The team adopted the principle of codesign when creating E-Heza, Rwanda's first point-of-care digital health record. The new digital tool serves the unique interests of all stakeholders. Nurses spend hours manually calculating Z-scores (standard deviations scores) to track a child's growth. A feature in E-Heza automatically calculates Z-scores when a nurse inputs a child's weight and height. This time-saving feature meets a real need of users and therefore may decrease the barriers to adoption.

Early prototypes were codesigned by nurses, mothers, designers, and health care administrators in brainstorming sessions. Testing sessions of digital prototypes invited feedback from stakeholders and helped to develop a health record that met the needs of users. E-Heza enables frontline workers to efficiently collect high-quality data; it can be used offline in areas of poor internet access; and it generates data reports that can be easily shared. This digital health solution has been piloted in nine health centers in Rwanda and may improve health outcomes in children by giving nurses a tool that helps them to perform health assessments on HIV-exposed infants.

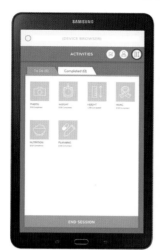
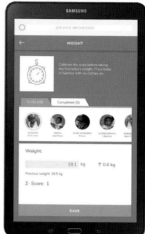

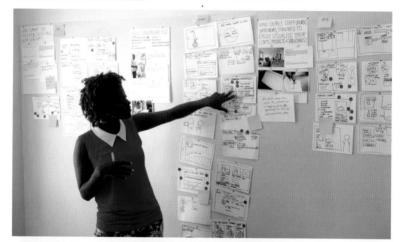

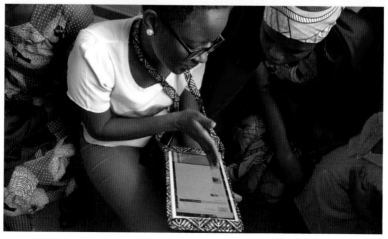

E-HEZA This tablet-based digital health record enables frontline health workers to efficiently capture measurements of height and weight and show mothers the data on their child's development.

READ MORE
→ greatergoodstudio.com/case-studies/the-ihangane-project/
→ ngopulse.org/article/2018/11/08/meet-non-profit-transforming-rwandan-healthcare

Clinical Trial Design

Everyone Included™ is a framework for health care innovation based on principles of mutual respect and inclusivity. It is the culmination of seven years of codesign with patients, caregivers, clinicians, technologists, and researchers at the Stanford University Medicine X program. The framework consists of a set of design and leadership principles intended to drive collaborative change in health care.

Optimal clinical trial design is needed for successful drug discovery and validation of new evidence-based treatments. The value of such work can be enhanced by developing greater partnerships with patients and the public in research data stewardship models; by creating productive policies on privacy, security, and ethics; and by setting research priorities and patient reported outcomes. Research shows that interventions and participant experiences can be improved by collaborating with patients and the public. Patient involvement in clinical trial design has been shown to generate a 500-fold return on investment and to speed new drugs to market by up to 2.5 years. In fact, many research funders are now recommending and requiring patient and public involvement in the design, conduct, and dissemination of health and social research studies.

This process is broadly termed "patient and public involvement" (PPI). Such involvement can occur throughout each stage of the research process, from designing a clinical trial to translating the results. But without clear PPI plans, researchers often focus on tokenistic engagement, or on involvement only in the recruitment or retention phases of research. Meaningful involvement and implementation of PPI requires thoughtful cultivation of partnerships and consistent engagement over time. Socially responsible and ethical research can be fostered through interconnected relationships between researchers and research partners (members of the public and patients), who provide a foundation for trustworthy "relational" engagements in research coproduction.

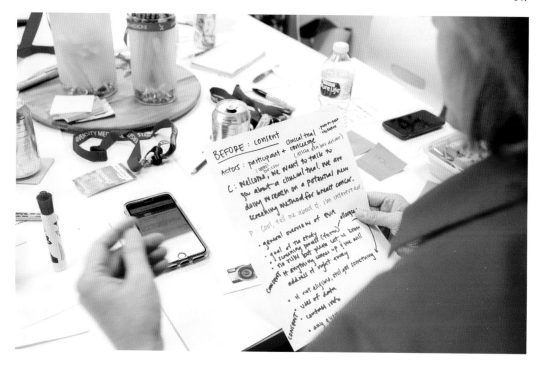

Codesigning clinical trials

Assemble a diverse team of patients and people who care for them, general members of the public, clinicians, allied health professionals, researchers (including epidemiologists and statisticians), and other specialists needed for the clinical trial area you intend to pursue.

Determine what question you want to answer. Use considerate leadership and Everyone Included™ design principles to identify the primary outcome measure and patient-centered outcome measures.

Work with patients and members of the public to codesign the methods and procedures that will be used in your trial. Consider ways to elicit and incorporate the goals, preferences, and values of participants.

Make prototypes of the experiences or methods that participants will encounter in your trial. Use the prototypes to iterate and improve these experiences or methods.

Prepare a patient and public involvement (PPI) plan for your study.

Present the study design, PPI plan, and protocol to other researchers, clinicians, and patient partners. Ask for honest feedback about the scientific validity of the design, its feasibility, and the patient experience.

Refine your design based on feedback.

Codesign in research involves flexible leadership between researcher, clinician, and patient to determine what types of services will meet the research question's most important goals, as defined by the team who can implement their plan together. This can be accomplished when clinical trial design is conducted with Everyone Included™.

A diverse team of breast cancer survivors, epidemiologists, cancer surgeons, machine learning/artificial intelligence experts, research nurses, research coordinators, evidence-based medicine experts, and public and patient partnership experts assembled around the shared goal of creating a clinical trial design for a novel digital breast cancer screening device.

Considerate leadership principles aim to flatten power hierarchies on diverse teams and to spotlight the unique skills and perspectives of each team member. These principles were used to create psychological safety and to elicit meaningful contributions from all team members. From the outset, these principles were shared with the team. The design process emphasized generating ideas over refinement or critique, especially in the early stages.

Using codesign research, the team engaged in two daylong design workshops, which guided participants through different parts of the clinical trial design process.

The first workshop focused on needs finding. After design facilitators provided a generic framework for journey mapping, the team was split into two balanced groups of stakeholders (patients, researchers, and technologists). The groups created detailed journey maps of either the current clinical trial process or the breast cancer screening experience. The groups regathered for presentation and discussion. This exercise revealed key points of frustration within the two processes and potential blind spots across the experiences of varied stakeholders. Knowledge of these frustration points and blind spots helped the team select which areas for improvement the clinical trial would address. The focus on the breast cancer screening process placed the clinical trial in a larger context and allowed for better integration of

the final protocol into the health care system. After the first workshop, the designers and patients on the team conducted follow-up interviews to answer further questions and synthesize insights.

The second workshop was held a month later and focused on the mechanics of the trial. The team was exposed to a diverse set of design methods, ranging from storyboarding to role-playing. The team used these methods to develop the specific procedures and interactions that would occur within the trial. The goal was to improve the patient experience throughout the trial process, from recruitment and enrollment to study completion.

Interactions through each stage of the proposed trial were prototyped and revised collaboratively, with a focus on the trial partic-ipant's experience, from the initial contact with the participant to a dissemination plan that would make the trial's results accessible to all stakeholders.

Finally, the proposed protocol was shared with an expert panel of outside and affiliated faculty biostatisticians and clinical trial experts to ensure the study was scientifically sound in capturing data in service of the primary and secondary outcomes.

Key findings included a strong desire among team members to see the following results: community among clinical trial participants; greater accessibility of and follow-up on post-trial results; and specific patient-centered outcomes focused on reducing anxiety and uncertainty around the breast cancer screening process. Another key finding was the benefit of discussing methodological limitations in nonthreatening ways and then working as a team to address them. One of the biggest takeaways came from reframing clinical trials: instead of viewing trials as tangential to a participant's care path, the team placed theml in the larger ecosystem of breast cancer screening and follow-up. Thus, this clinical trial design became a new way of achieving broader health care goals, such as empowering participants to build community and become more informed, and setting the stage for greater participation in research. These insights were achieved by including everyone in clinical trial design.

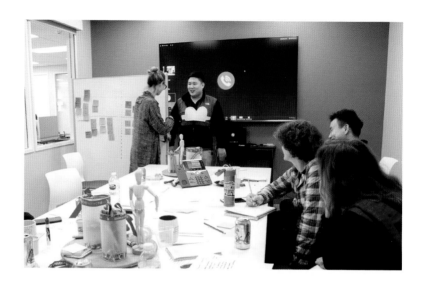

Stanford Medicine X Everyone Included™ clinical trial design team, Stanford University School of Medicine: Larry Chu, MD (PI, researcher, epidemiologist), Urvi Gupta and Dominick Zheng (designers), Liza Bernstein and Alicia Staley (breast cancer survivors, patient partners), Haythem Ali, MD (breast cancer surgeon), Martha Tingle, RN (research nurse), Timothy Lee (research coordinator), Amy Price, PhD (evidence-based medicine specialist), Dara Rouholiman (machine learning, artificial intelligence specialist), Kim Smuga-Otto (science communication specialist)

WORKING BETTER TOGETHER (above) Interdisciplinary stakeholders assemble to prototype specific experiences of the proposed clinical trial through role-playing. Researchers, patients, technologists, and designers merged expertise using the Everyone Included™ codesign and collaboration framework. By engaging with a diverse set of experts, a team can design a clinical trial protocol that elevates the participant experience while remaining statistically valid. Photos: Golnaz Shahmirzadi for Stanford Medicine X

READ MORE

Cribb, A., and Gewirtz, S. "New Welfare Ethics and the Remaking of Identities in an Era of User Involvement." *Globalisation, Societies and Education* 10, no. 4 (2012): 507–17.

Evans, S., Corley, M., Corrie, M., Costley, K., and Donald, C. "Evaluating Services in Partnership with Older People: Exploring the Role of Community Researchers." *Working with Older People* 15, no. 1 (2011): 26–33.

Fleurence, R., Selby, J. V., Odom-Walker, K., et al. "How the Patient-Centered Outcomes Research Institute Is Engaging Patients and Others in Shaping Its Research Agenda." *Health Affairs* 32, no. 2 (2013): 393–400.

Levitan, B., Getz, K., Eisenstein, E., et al. "Assessing the Financial Value of Patient Engagement: A Quantitative Approach from CTTI's Patient Groups and Clinical Trials Project." *Therapeutic Innovation & Regulatory Science.* 2017: 1–10.

Mockford, C., Staniszewska, S., Griffiths, F., and Herron-Marx, S. "The Impact of Patient and Pubic Involvement on UK NHS Health Care: A Systematic Review." *International Journal for Quality in Health Care* 24, no. 1 (2012): 28–38.

Research NIfH. *Patient and Public Involvement in Health and Social Care Research: A Handbook for Researchers.* London: National Institute for Health Research, 2010.

Shippee, N.D., Domecq Garces J.P., Prutsky Lopez G.J., et al. "Patient and Service User Engagement in Research: A Systematic Review and Synthesized Framework." *Health Expectations* 18, no. 5 (2015): 1151–66.

Stanford Medicine: Medicine X. "Everyone Included: Improving Health Care Together." Richards, T., Schroter, S., Price, A., and Godlee, F. "Better Together: Patient Partnership in Medical Journals." *BMJ* (Clinical research ed.) 362 (2018): k3798.

→ www.everyoneincluded.org. Accessed February 1, 2016.

Informed Consent

At Vanderbilt University Medical Center in Nashville, Tennessee, researchers in surgical ethics and human-centered legal design initiated a comprehensive study of the informed consent process for surgical procedures. Their process, which includes background preparation, interviewing, observing, prototyping, and testing, provides a useful model for how to deeply explore a design challenge over a sustained period.

The project originated from related research involving interviews with surgeons, anesthesiologists, nurses, and patients across the U.S. about the process of obtaining permission from people to perform surgery (informed consent). After conducting additional research, the team identified a group of gatekeepers at the medical center—representatives in perioperative administration, hospital general counsel, risk management, patient affairs, and information technology. Meetings with these gatekeepers helped secure guidance and buy-in from across the hospital.

Next, the team talked with patients and clinicians about the informed consent process. Because surgical procedures are major life events with which people have little or no prior experience, many individuals reported having difficulty picking through the fine print of the consent document; some would prefer a guided experience with clinician assistance or a more interactive document. Clinicians valued a streamlined process that minimizes unnecessary work, and they pointed out that the increasing burdens of medical documentation detract from face-to-face discussions and diminish the bond of trust with patients.

In the project at Vanderbilt, an immersive design boot camp was followed by two academic courses—one in systems design (School of Engineering) and the other in legal problem-solving (Law School). These courses culminated in open ideation and prototyping sessions. The next steps in this ongoing project are to select a testing strategy and determine metrics for successful implementation.

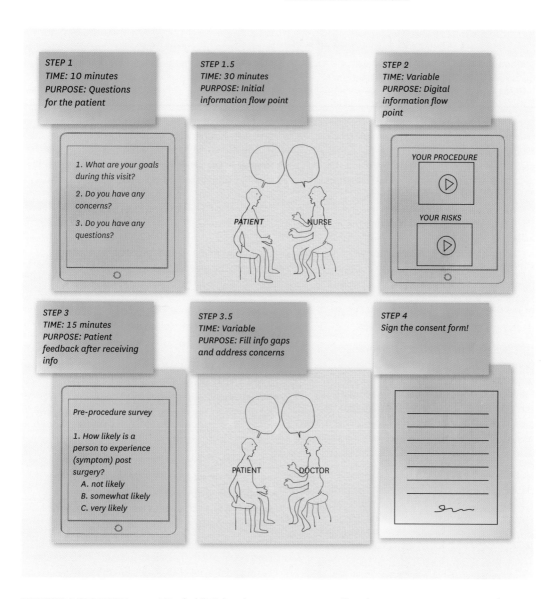

MAPPING A PROCESS Teams at Vanderbilt University Medical Center applied design thinking to the process of informed consent. They mapped out new user journeys and designed simple mock-ups of app interfaces. The informed consent process shown here includes a sketch for a digital app and conversations between patients and clinicians. Color coding helps clarify the process: blue for digital interactions, yellow for face-to-face interactions, and green for identifying the steps.

CONTRIBUTORS Alexander Langerman, MD, SM, FACS, Associate Professor of Otolaryngology, Director of the Surgical Analytics Lab, and Faculty of the Center for Biomedical Ethics and Society and the Institute for Surgery and Engineering, Vanderbilt University Medical Center, Nashville, TN; Caitlin Moon, JD, MA, Adjunct Professor of Law, Director of Innovation Design of the Program in Law and Innovation, Director of the PoLI Institute, Vanderbilt University Law School, Nashville, TN

BACKGROUND RESEARCH Interviews demonstrated a disconnect between patients' understanding of the surgical process and clinicians' assumptions about patient understanding. Furthermore, although clinicians felt that they had meaningful discussions with people about surgical procedures, they believed that the informed consent document (the official permission slip signed by the patient) did not enable or adequately represent the communication and decision-making process surrounding "true" informed consent.

Additional research on case law and the ethical basis of informed consent revealed the normative expectations and goals of informed consent. Research also showed that people were not always truly aware of the details despite consenting to procedures. Informed consent discussions frequently leaned more toward disclosure than toward the more desirable model of shared decision-making.

GATEKEEPER INTERVIEWS Rather than seeking permission to "change informed consent," the team structured their meetings with adminstrative leaders as interviews for building empathy by learning from their experiences and unique knowledge. This phase of the project was framed as a fact-finding mission about informed consent at Vanderbilt University Medical Center.

USER INTERVIEWS Next, the team reached out to patients and clinicians working in the perioperative environment—these are the users who would "touch" an informed consent document, bringing diverse perspectives to the process. People described informed consent documents as intimidating forms full of legal terms. These same patients were surprised to discover some of the content of the document once they did read it. Conversely, doctors communicated with patients about the risks, benefits, and alternatives of surgery (the essential elements of informed consent) on a daily basis, and described the document signing as "checking a box" rather than explaining that it was a significant aid to the doctor-patient relationship. Nurses noted the one-way nature of the document—it disclosed information but did not engage the patient as a partner in the process. (For example, expectations that individuals will participate in their own recovery are not prompted.) Clinicians, risk managers, and general counsel all saw a "good informed consent" as ensuring that patients are making an educated decision consistent with their goals and as protecting patients through accurate documentation of the plan of care (e.g., the operation to be performed and on which body part). The consent document itself has multiple subsections, each serving a different function in the process—yet not all aspects of an ideal informed consent are represented.

RESEARCH BOOT CAMP Armed with these insights, a research team comprising students in law, management, engineering, and medicine convened for a design boot camp. To save time and achieve focus, this workshop emphasized just one element of the problem: "How might we improve the patient experience?" The boot camp began with interactive education on steps in the design thinking process (empathize, define, ideate, and prototype), which the team then practiced in small groups with invited patients and clinicians. In addition to generating ideas and involving users, the boot camp built cross-disciplinary cohesion within the team and provided basic design training.

FIELD RESEARCH Academic coursework in systems design and legal problem-solving allowed for study in greater depth. Students made field visits to clinical environments (outpatient clinic, preoperative holding areas, and emergency department) to observe the informed consent process and talk with clinicians and patients. Both classes compiled and shared field notes with the research team.

OPEN PROTOTYPE The classes culminated in open ideation and prototyping sessions with stakeholders, allowing for real-time feedback and rapid refinement of ideas.

VETTING AND TESTING The decision to focus on the patient experience was deliberate, but it also resulted in solutions that would not satisfy all stakeholders. Many of the prototypes would have greatly increased the documentation burden on clinicians, and/or they relied heavily on multimedia that supplanted direct doctor–patient communication. The document was at risk of being overdesigned and of yielding a process that would not realistically fit into clinical workflow. To this end, a reality check phase would need to be conducted to explore the creation of more modest but still meaningful changes. The absence of constraints early in the process allowed for free idea generation, and these ideas would now be considered within the overall system in which the document would need to perform.

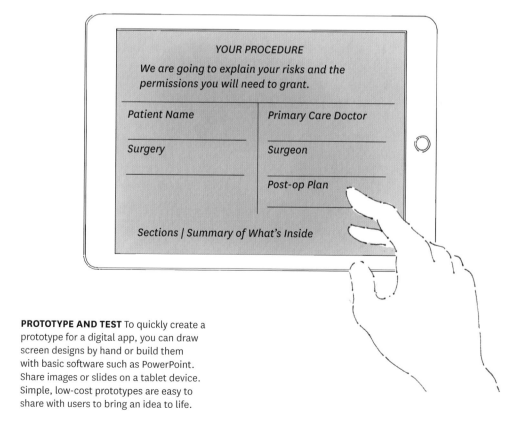

PROTOTYPE AND TEST To quickly create a prototype for a digital app, you can draw screen designs by hand or build them with basic software such as PowerPoint. Share images or slides on a tablet device. Simple, low-cost prototypes are easy to share with users to bring an idea to life.

Visual Health History

Twelve million people in the U.S. are misdiagnosed or remain undiagnosed each year. A major cause of this problem is broken communication. People with invisible symptoms or complex histories are often misunderstood or disbelieved by their doctors.

   Katie McCurdy has experienced this dynamic firsthand. As a long-time autoimmune patient who is also a designer, she started creating health history timelines and symptom maps to explain her story. These visual tools helped her communicate more clearly while enabling her doctors to understand her story without digging through the EHR. This experience inspired McCurdy to create Pictal Health, a service that brings visual communication to patients and doctors.

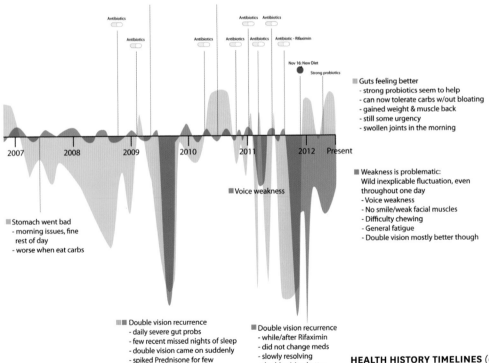

HEALTH HISTORY TIMELINES (details) These temporal graphs show how a person's treatments, symptoms, and life events overlap. Seeing events laid out in this way is illuminating for both patients and doctors. Design: Katie McCurdy, Pictal Health

Meet Darren (not his real name), who had suffered symptoms for most of his life with no satisfactory diagnosis or relief. Along with having sharp abdominal pain, he'd been seeing blood in the toilet every day for almost two years. With each new doctor he saw, he had to start over and revisit failed treatments. He was extremely frustrated—and dangerously anemic.

Darren came to his first meeting with McCurdy holding a four-page, single-spaced printout of his health history—comprehensive but difficult to parse. Together, they plotted out the major points on a large hand-drawn timeline, and McCurdy asked Darren many questions. She asked him to draw how his body felt when he was feeling bad or feeling good. They created a shared document that stated what treatments had been tried and what diagnoses had been ruled out. After the first meeting, McCurdy created a refined visual timeline that showed how Darren's symptoms had unfolded in relation to key tests, diagnoses, and treatments.

After making a few revisions to his health timeline, Darren was ready for his first appointment with a new gastroenterologist. He practiced talking through his story and brought extra copies to leave with the staff. The doctor was very receptive to the visuals and gave him plenty of time to talk through his story. Because his health history and past treatment attempts were easy for the doctor to absorb, Darren was able to avoid having to repeat ineffective treatments. In subsequent appointments, he noticed that doctors and staff would show up to his room holding printouts of his health timeline and summary.

As a designer, McCurdy learned the importance of each step in the process, from having the initial conversation to organizing the health summary, creating a visual timeline, and preparing for the doctor visit. Talking through their stories primes people to recall details more accurately. This process has helped Darren and other patients feel heard. The visual format lets them externalize their complex backgrounds, freeing them from keeping every detail in their minds. The graphics help doctors absorb what the person is telling them.

McCurdy has continued to work with other individuals with complex health histories—including Lyme, autoimmune, and other conditions—and is continually refining her process and bringing it to more patients and doctors.

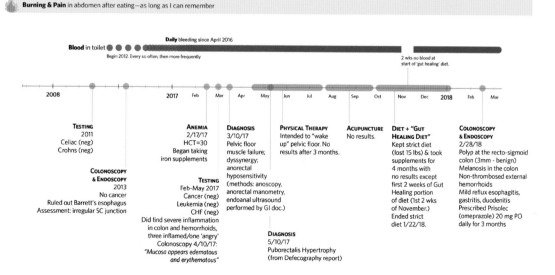

Burning & Pain in abdomen after eating—as long as I can remember

Blood in toilet — **Daily** bleeding since April 2016

Begin 2012. Every so often, then more frequently

2 wks no blood at start of 'gut healing' diet.

| 2008 | 2017 | Feb | Mar | Apr | May | Jun | Jul | Aug | Sep | Oct | Nov | Dec | 2018 | Feb | Mar |

TESTING
2011
Celiac (neg)
Crohns (neg)

COLONOSCOPY & ENDOSCOPY
2013
No cancer
Ruled out Barrett's esophagus
Assessment: irregular SC junction

ANEMIA
2/17/17
HCT=30
Began taking iron supplements

TESTING
Feb–May 2017
Cancer (neg)
Leukemia (neg)
CHF (neg)
Did find severe inflammation in colon and hemorrhoids, three inflamed/one 'angry'
Colonoscopy 4/10/17:
"Mucosa appears edematous and erythematous"

DIAGNOSIS
3/10/17
Pelvic floor muscle failure; dyssynergy; anorectal hyposensitivity (methods: anoscopy, anorectal manometry, endoanal ultrasound performed by GI doc.)

DIAGNOSIS
5/10/17
Puborectalis Hypertrophy (from Defecography report)

PHYSICAL THERAPY
Intended to "wake up" pelvic floor. No results after 3 months.

ACUPUNCTURE
No results.

DIET + "GUT HEALING DIET"
Kept strict diet (lost 15 lbs) & took supplements for 4 months with no results except first 2 weeks of Gut Healing portion of diet (1st 2 wks of November.)
Ended strict diet 1/22/18.

COLONOSCOPY & ENDOSCOPY
2/28/18
Polyp at the recto-sigmoid colon (3mm - benign)
Melanosis in the colon
Non-thrombosed external hemorrhoids
Mild reflux esophagitis, gastritis, duodenitis
Prescribed Prisolec (omeprazole) 20 mg PO daily for 3 months

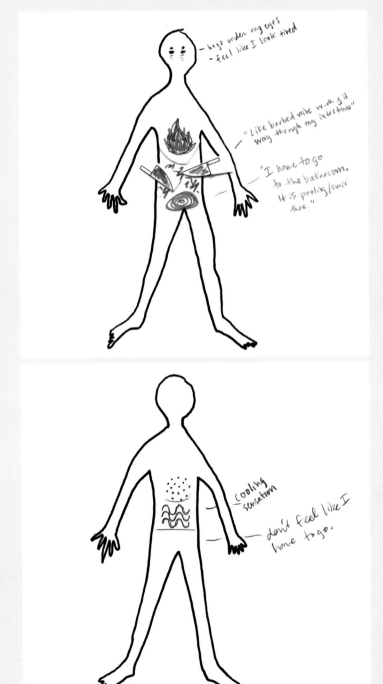

SYMPTOM MAPS Simple diagrams help patients communicate their experiences of positive and negative states. Design: Katie McCurdy, Pictal Health

Symptoms

What my symptoms look like when they flare up—
often due to a chemical exposure

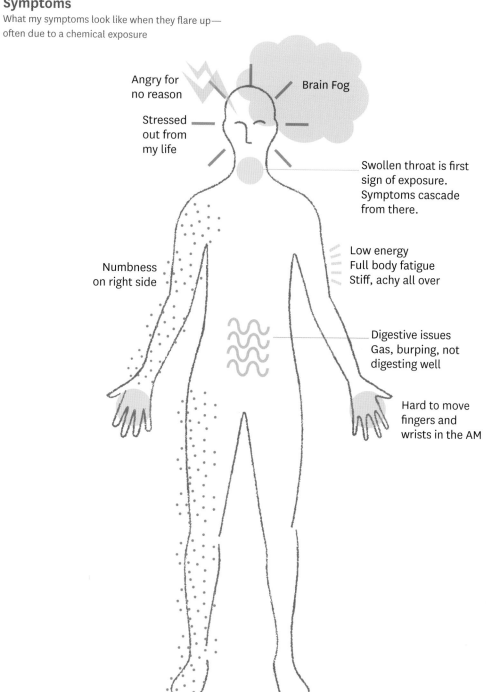

Angry for
no reason

Brain Fog

Stressed
out from
my life

Swollen throat is first
sign of exposure.
Symptoms cascade
from there.

Numbness
on right side

Low energy
Full body fatigue
Stiff, achy all over

Digestive issues
Gas, burping, not
digesting well

Hard to move
fingers and
wrists in the AM

Shared Decision-Making

Much health care communication and decision making fails to acknowledge and address people's situation. Ms. B has type 2 diabetes and a blood sugar level above the target set by clinical guidelines. Her clinician would likely tell her that she needs to pay more attention to her diet, get more exercise, and take medications. Ms. B would hear this information and accept the prescription, but her true decision making would happen later, when she decides whether or not to fill the prescription, or take it as it was prescribed, or refill it. In her internal decision-making process, she might consider issues that didn't come up in her visit with the clinician, such as perceived need and benefit (*why am I taking this?*), importance (*can I deal with this right now?*), cost (*can I afford this?*), and impact on other life aspects (*will this change the way I look? my sleep? my sex life?*).

The effect of her decision will show up in a lab test measuring her blood sugar levels. If the numbers are still too high, her clinician will likely suggest an intensification of therapy in the form of an increased dosage or an additional medication. Those other issues that Ms. B considered may never come up because the clinician doesn't ask, and Ms. B may not consider them relevant or perhaps fears being judged. If Ms. B's blood sugar level continues to exceed the target set by guidelines, she may earn the label "noncompliant," which implies moral failure and can lead Ms. B's clinician and the clinical system to pull away from Ms. B's care.

This disconnect is a problem at the heart of patient–clinician communication. Shared decision-making addresses the issue by providing a framework for conversation, often in the form of a tool, that both parties can use to find a common way forward that makes practical, intellectual, and emotional sense: practical, meaning what someone can do and make work in their life; intellectual, meaning informed by evidence and clinical knowledge; and emotional, meaning responsive to the feelings generated.

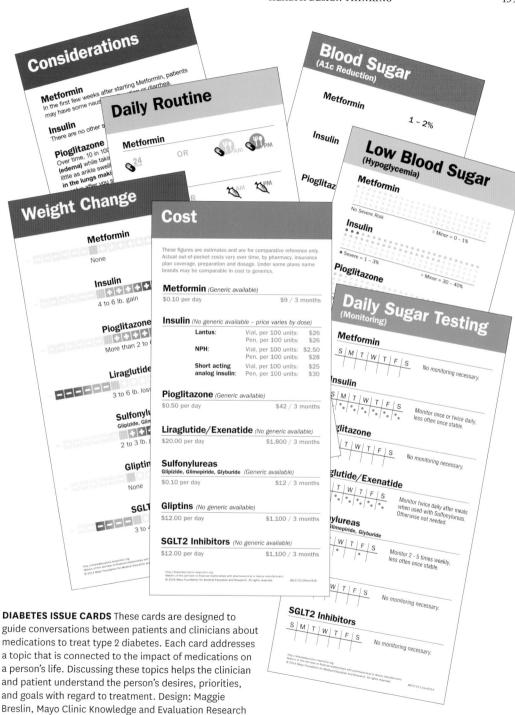

DIABETES ISSUE CARDS These cards are designed to guide conversations between patients and clinicians about medications to treat type 2 diabetes. Each card addresses a topic that is connected to the impact of medications on a person's life. Discussing these topics helps the clinician and patient understand the person's desires, priorities, and goals with regard to treatment. Design: Maggie Breslin, Mayo Clinic Knowledge and Evaluation Research (KER) Unit, Mayo Clinic Illustration and Design

Consider this conversation where a decision tool is used. A ninety-year-old man and his primary care doctor meet and use a tool for diabetes medications. The man is a widower preparing to move into a nursing home.

Clinician displays set of cards.

CLINICIAN Which of these issues would you be interested in discussing?

Patient selects Weight Change.

Clinician expresses surprise.

PATIENT You know I'm moving into a nursing home, Doc, and those places are filled with single ladies. I've got to look my best.

Clinician laughs. Patient points to Exenatide, a drug that offers possible weight loss. Clinician points patient toward the Daily Routine card.

CLINICIAN Now, Exanatide is an injectable.

PATIENT That's no problem. The nurses give you your shots in the nursing home, and they are pretty cute too.

Clinician laughs again.

CLINICIAN Okay. Well, let's give it a try.

In this interaction, the tool has helped surface some issues about the patient's life that have an impact on the decisions he and the clinician will make together.

The process of creating shared decision-making tools benefits from the collaborative efforts of a number of disciplines. The teams at Mayo Clinic's Knowledge and Evaluation Research (KER) Unit and The Patient Revolution bring together clinicians, designers, clinical researchers, subject matter experts, and patients in the process of building tools together. To begin, the designers conduct observations of clinical visits to understand the current state of conversations and get a sense of the issues that are likely to be important to doctors and patients. The researchers and clinicians review the medical literature to identify the options, evidence, recommendations, and uncertainties that could become content for the tool. The designers then create prototypes of the tool. The prototypes represent hypotheses about which topics and flows will best support productive dialogue. These prototypes are evaluated in the clinical setting, with actual clinicians and patients using them as they work through real situations. The designers and researchers look for changes in the conversation, observing whether issues and topics that previously went unaddressed are now part of the discussion.

Because these tools are intended to support dialogue during the clinical visit, they must address the constraints of traditional clinical spaces. Tools can be digital or physical. Digital tools are easier to update and distribute and may accommodate integration into the electronic health record, but they may require clinicians and patients to reorient to the computer, depending on the space they find themselves in. Physical tools, such as cards, have a form that reinforces the conversational goal and integrates easily into any space, but keeping the evidence updated and distributing the product can be more challenging.

The conversations created when using a shared decision-making tool will not all look the same. The conversations do not follow a script. Some people might look at a video of a conversation where a tool is used and find it lacking. They might have advice for the clinician and patient about what they should have mentioned or how they should have talked about an issue. However, the purpose of shared decision-making is not to create a perfect conversation. It is to help these people address a situation and, ideally, build their relationship so that the connection and the trust spill into their next encounter.

The tools are by design incomplete. The tools need a clinician and a patient to fill in the spaces with the specific challenges and opportunities represented by the clinical situation and the person's life. Shared decision-making tools thus embody a larger goal: to reconnect clinicians and patients in productive conversations.

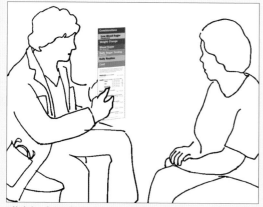

Clinician introduces tool to discuss diabetes medications.

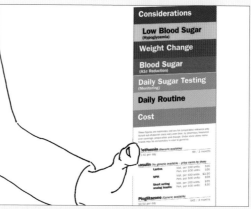

Clinician asks, "Which issue would you like to start with?"

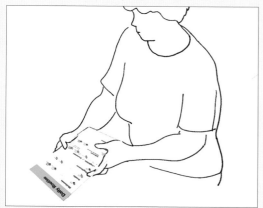

Patient reviews a card and considers a medication.

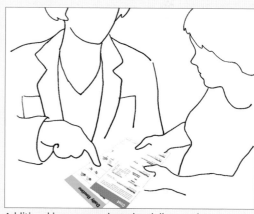

Additional issues are selected and discussed.

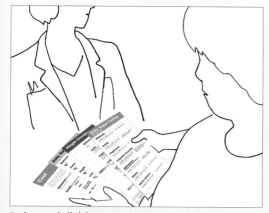

Patient and clinician narrow in on an option.

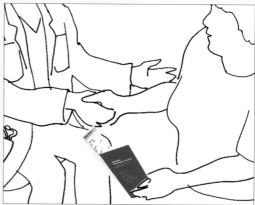

Patient and clinician agree on a care plan.

Personalized Asthma Care

"In a fifteen-minute clinic visit, we can only treat from the neck on down to the diaphragm." This statement was the spark that led Mandeep Jassal and Christy Sadreameli, two pediatric pulmonologists from the Johns Hopkins Children's Center, to approach the Center for Social Design at Maryland Institute College of Art (MICA). A team of designers worked with clinicians, parents of children with asthma, and other community stakeholders to learn how families in Baltimore City experience asthma and design ways to better connect the clinic experience to patients' day-to-day lives.

One in seven kids in Baltimore has asthma—that's almost twice the national average. It is also a major health justice issue in the city, because black children are significantly more likely than white children to have asthma and to be hospitalized for complications. Asthma is the kind of challenge that design thinking is well suited to explore.

To begin the project, the team created case studies of existing asthma interventions in Baltimore and took note of key themes. The team also conducted ethnographic observations in a pediatric asthma clinic, and at public events around Baltimore City, like community organizing meetings and a local health exposition. After building a solid background about how people are currently addressing asthma, the team conducted interviews with two adolescent asthma patients, ten caregivers, two community advocates, three social workers, three doctors, and one nurse.

The insights the team learned from these stakeholders formed the basis of a brainstorming session with caregivers, physicians, social workers, and others who work with asthma. The goal of this session was to imagine ideas without constraints—this process is "idea generative" rather than "idea selective." The session produced over two hundred ideas, ranging from having kids use Snapchat to show their families that they took their meds, to a "golden inhaler trophy" that recognizes the efforts of all-star caregivers. At the end of the session, each participant received five stickers for "voting" for the ideas they would most like see come to life. The top-voted ideas got a chance to become real interventions through the prototyping process.

Insights: pediatric asthma care

Success relies on team effort, and kids are part of that team.

Clinicians tend to primarily engage caregivers in conversations about asthma, leaving the child out of the conversation. We asked: How might we shift asthma education from instruction to a conversation?

The exam room feels disconnected from real life in the home.

Knowing about the patient's home life not only builds trust and collaboration between clinician and caregiver but also allows the clinician to give better health care advice for patients. We asked: How might we help clinicians understand the lives of their patients and their families?

Being a caregiver is hard work, but not everyone has the support they need.

Clinicians may not always know what the caregiver's support systems are like, and that may affect the quality of trust and collaboration between clinician and caregiver. We asked: How might we create opportunities for caregivers to share their needs with clinicians?

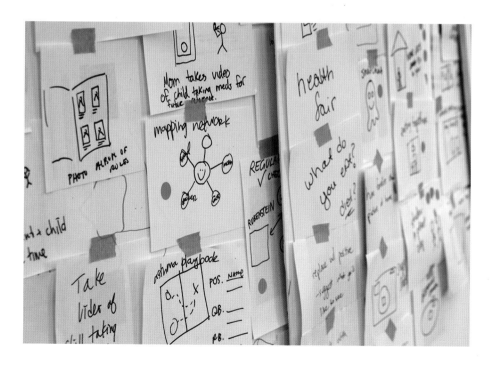

EARLY PROTOTYPES The first versions used materials like pencil sketches, Legos, and cotton swabs. One idea was to have caregivers pair up to support each other. The prototype the team created, inspired by "best friends" jewelry for kids, was a set of two necklaces, each one representing half of a lung, that caregivers could wear to remind themselves that they aren't alone. The first prototype was made with Play-Doh and yarn—not gold. That's good, because this idea didn't ultimately move forward.

IMPLEMENTATION The team identified which prototypes best addressed the project's key insights and worked on refining them. During the final group studio session, clinicians and caregivers interacted with multiple prototypes and gave their feedback. Ultimately, three ideas from these sessions became real programs that are being implemented in the clinic. These programs will evolve and adapt as they are used more—that's the magic of prototyping.

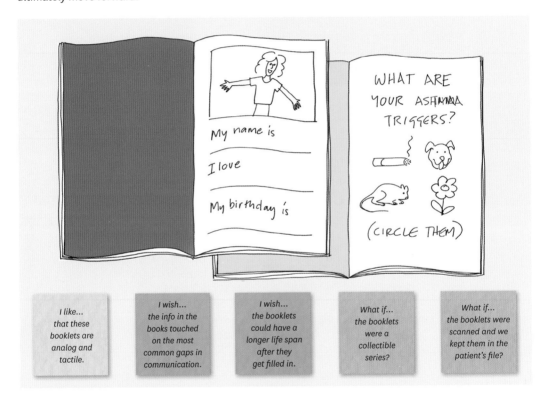

I like...
that these
booklets are
analog and
tactile.

I wish...
the info in the
books touched
on the most
common gaps in
communication.

I wish...
the booklets
could have a
longer life span
after they
get filled in.

What if...
the booklets
were a
collectible
series?

What if...
the booklets were
scanned and we
kept them in the
patient's file?

I LIKE/I WISH/WHAT IF? A good framework for gathering feedback on prototypes is called "I like/I wish/What if?" Participants write what they like about the prototype, what they wish the prototype could do, and ideas they want to add.

MICA Center for Social Design: Design team: Franki Abraham, Katie Mancher, Delaney Todd, Kimmy Tsai, Amanda Velez-Cortes, Maddie Wolf, and Christina Yoo; Faculty advisors: Becky Slogeris and Ashley Eberhart. Partner: Johns Hopkins Children's Center: Mandeep Jassal, Christy Sadreameli, Hilary Heslep, Helen Hughes, Arlene Butz, Cassie Lewis-Land, and Peter Mogayzel

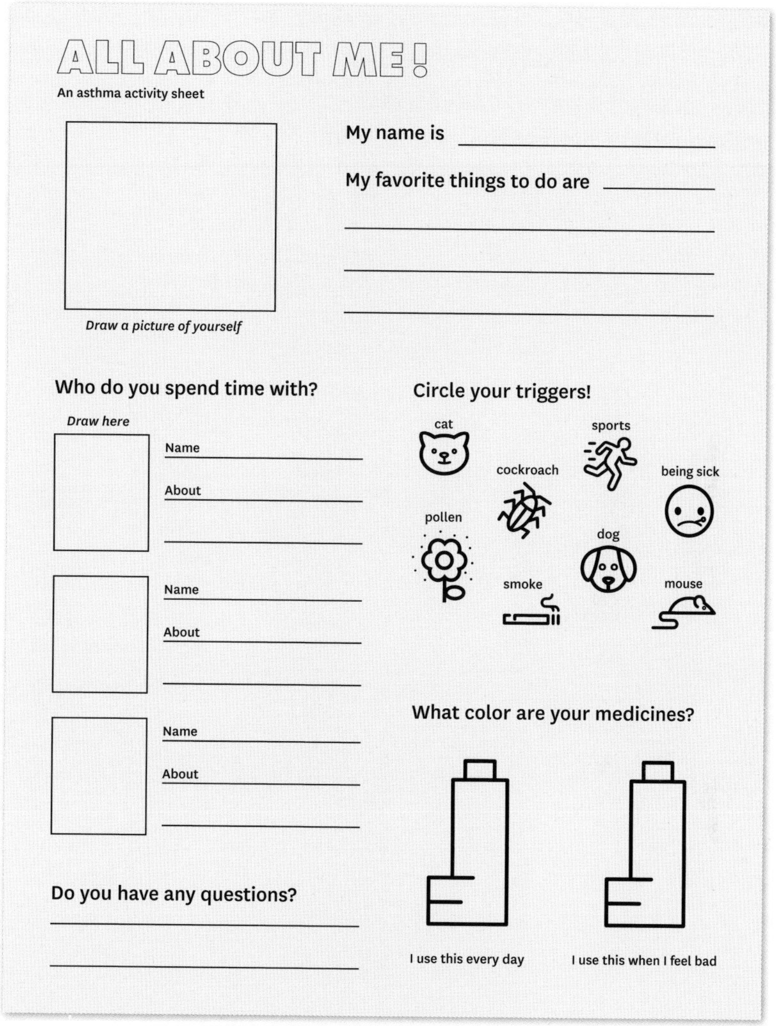

ALL ABOUT ME!

An asthma activity sheet

Draw a picture of yourself

My name is _____

My favorite things to do are _____

_____

_____

_____

Who do you spend time with?

Draw here

Name _____

About _____

_____

Name _____

About _____

_____

Name _____

About _____

Circle your triggers!

cat   sports

cockroach   being sick

pollen

dog

smoke   mouse

What color are your medicines?

Do you have any questions?

_____

_____

_____

I use this every day   I use this when I feel bad

Asthma activity sheet

Design: Kimmy Tsai

WHAT A worksheet for children gives clinicians a better sense of a patient's life outside the clinic and of what the patient knows about their asthma care.

HOW In the waiting room, children complete this fun activity about themselves, their homes, their family, and their asthma care. The worksheet helps engage them during otherwise "dead time"—and their caregiver may appreciate the break so that they can fill out their own pre-visit paperwork.

WHY Clinicians can use the worksheet to meaningfully engage children in care conversations. For instance, the drawing prompt "Who do you spend the most time with?" can start a conversation about the allocation of medication roles in the household.

Sharing feedback at every stage is critical in prototyping. It helps you build on what works—and discard what doesn't—before you've gone too far and gotten attached to an idea.

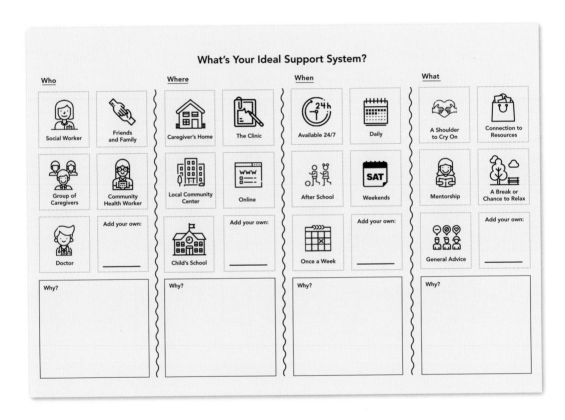

Caregiver-designed support system   Design: Amanda Velez-Cortes

WHAT A visual decision-making aid that social workers use to spark dialogue with caregivers about what support they need to manage the child's asthma

HOW In a meeting with a social worker, caregivers select icons representing the support they need: who (nurse, peers), what (advice, childcare), where (home, library), and when (weekends, 24/7). The tool helps them design a support system that could work best for them.

WHY This conversation aid helps caregivers design support systems they'd actually want to use. If the type of resource they prefer (such as "a hotline for medical advice that's available 24/7") already exists, the social worker can link them to it. If it doesn't, the clinic can try to start it.

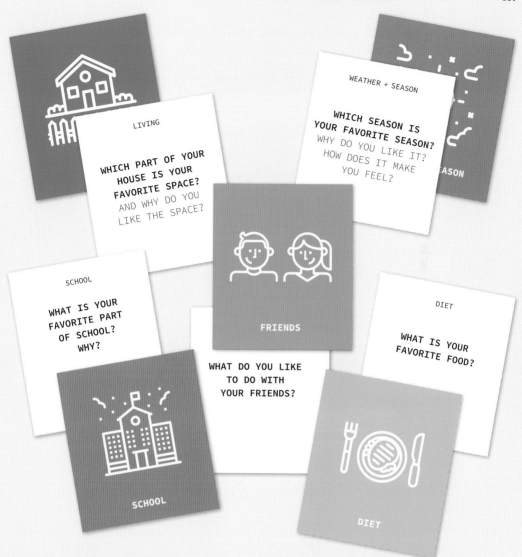

Conversation starter pack

Design: Christina Yoo

WHAT A deck of cards with kid-friendly prompts that help build a relationship of trust and collaboration among clinicians, caregivers, and patients.

HOW On the way to the exam room, or during the first few minutes of an appointment, a clinician holds out the deck of cards and asks their pediatric patient to select one. The quick, easy conversation prompts in the deck facilitate relationship-building among clinicians, caregivers, and patients.

WHY Clinic visits go fast, but relationships take time to build. These mini-prompts offer a practical way for clinicians to connect on a personal level with their patients and caregivers, thereby building a foundation for trust and collaboration despite tough time constraints.

READ MORE Ashley Eberhart *et al.*, "Using a Human-centered Design Approach for Collaborative Decision-making in Pediatric Asthma Care," *Public Health*, → doi.org/10.1016/j.puhe.2019.03.004.

Smoke-Free Homes

Cigarette smoking is the largest preventable cause of death and disease in the United States, killing over 480,000 people a year. More than 41,000 of these deaths are due to exposure to secondhand smoke. Like most public health agencies, the Baltimore City Health Department used to lean heavily on traditional approaches to helping people quit smoking, such as making presentations about health risks at community meetings and distributing brochures with additional facts and resources. But these methods alone were not making the impact the health department wanted to see.

After deciding they needed a new approach, the Baltimore City Health Department partnered with the Center for Social Design at the Maryland Institute College of Art (MICA) to rethink how they engage residents around smoking. Using design thinking methods, students met with health professionals to better understand the problem, interviewed Baltimore families to gain new insights, and facilitated design workshops to generate ideas and prototypes.

The research and brainstorming resulted in HealthiAir, a pop-up event that supports families in creating smoke-free comfort zones in their homes by helping them identify practical ways to get started and connecting them to resources. Instead of sitting in an audience listening to a person in the front of the room talk at them, participants move through five stations that feature different prompts and activities aligned with the stages of health behavior change.

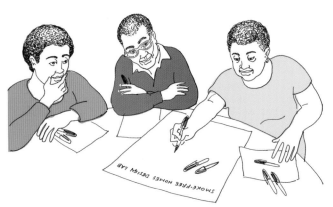

"I feel good about making changes in my household."

"I would recommend this program to my husband to get him to quit smoking."

PARTICIPANT FEEDBACK

Changing health behavior

1. SHARING STORIES (Precontemplation) Creating an open space for sharing and connecting with others about how smoking has affected you personally

2. EXPLORING THE OPPORTUNITIES (Contemplation) Imagining, through drawing or writing, what your ideal smoke-free comfort zone would look like and how it would feel

3. ACCEPTING THE CHALLENGE (Preparation) Discovering the benefits and challenges of creating your smoke-free comfort zone and identifying your first step by signing a family pledge

4. CONTINUING THE PROCESS (Action) Celebrating where you are on the journey and finding ways to keep yourself on track by creating House Promises (realistic and achievable steps made by families to create and maintain smoke-free comfort zones)

5. SUPPORTING THE JOURNEY (Maintenance) Connecting you to additional resources that will ultimately help you quit smoking and give you the opportunity to continue sharing your experience by becoming a HealthiAir Community Advocate

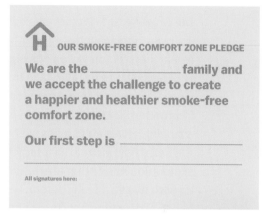

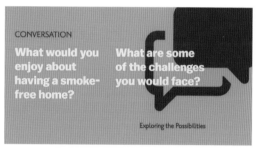

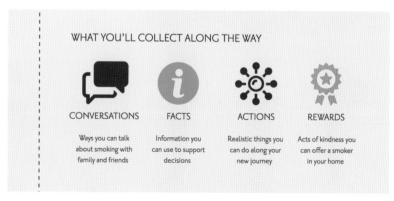

Project team: MICA Center for Social Design: Mike Weikert, director; Becky Slogeris, faculty adviser; Denise Shanté Brown and Smile Indias, design strategists. Design team: Amanda Buck, Hayley Frazier, Mihoshi Fukushima, Jenny Hung, Christy Tang, Naeeme Mohammadi. Partner: Baltimore City Health Department.

Puberty Education

The Growing Girls Project was born of a desire for every girl to grow up loving and accepting herself fully. In service to this mission, researchers at Johns Hopkins Bloomberg School of Public Health and designers at the Maryland Institute College of Art (MICA) created innovative puberty education tools that are designed to help young girls understand, connect with, appreciate, and respect their changing selves and bodies as they enter puberty.

These tools include an interactive activity book and a self-exploration mirror that are designed as gifts to young girls, ages eight to twelve, ideally before, or just as, they show the first signs of pubertal development (breast buds and/or pubic hair). These tools were created in response to the experiences, recommendations, and feedback of young people in Baltimore City.

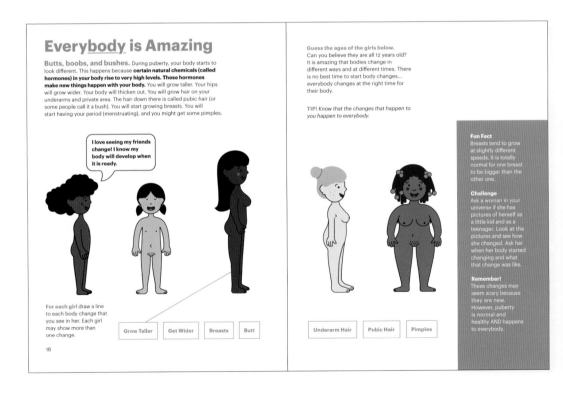

Everybody is Amazing

Butts, boobs, and bushes. During puberty, your body starts to look different. This happens because **certain natural chemicals (called hormones) in your body rise to very high levels. These hormones make new things happen with your body.** You will grow taller. Your hips will grow wider. Your body will thicken out. You will grow hair on your underarms and private area. The hair down there is called pubic hair (or some people call it a bush). You will start growing breasts. You will start having your period (menstruating), and you might get some pimples.

Guess the ages of the girls below. Can you believe they are all 12 years old? It is amazing that bodies change in different ways and at different times. There is no best time to start body changes... everybody changes at the right time for their body.

TIP! *Know that the changes that happen to you happen to everybody.*

> I love seeing my friends change! I know my body will develop when it is ready.

Fun Fact
Breasts tend to grow at slightly different speeds. It is totally normal for one breast to be bigger than the other one.

Challenge
Ask a woman in your universe if she has pictures of herself as a little kid and as a teenager. Look at the pictures and see how she changed. Ask her when her body started changing and what that change was like.

Remember!
These changes may seem scary because they are new. However, puberty is normal and healthy AND happens to everybody.

For each girl draw a line to each body change that you see in her. Each girl may show more than one change.

| Grow Taller | Get Wider | Breasts | Butt |

| Underarm Hair | Pubic Hair | Pimples |

18

Project leads: Ann Herbert, PhD, Johns Hopkins Bloomberg School of Public Health, and Jennifer Cole Phillips, MICA. Project Designers: Katja Fluekiger, Kavya Barthwal, Dan Spurgin, Shivani Parasnis, Andrew Peters, Brooke Thyng, and Jarrett Fuller. Photography: Dan Spurgin

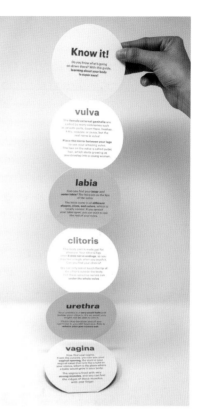

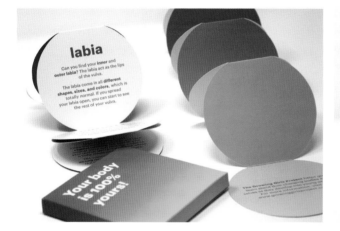

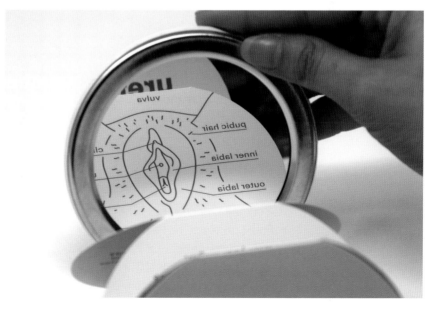

Demand for Chlorhexidine

From 1990 to 2017, the number of newborns who died within their first month of life decreased by nearly 50%. However, in 2017, still over 2.5 million newborns died within their first month of life. The majority of these deaths could have been prevented with simple, affordable interventions. Sepsis (infection) in newborns often occurs via the umbilical cord. Chlorhexidine is an antiseptic applied to the cord stump after birth. When used in high-risk settings on the first day of life, chlorhexidine can reduce neonatal mortality by over 20%. Chlorhexidine is low-cost (less than 25 cents per dose), simple to use, and easy to manufacture. Yet, in high-risk settings, chlorhexidine still isn't widely used. The U.S. Agency for International Development (USAID), in partnership with Dalberg Design, applied a design thinking approach to spark demand for this lifesaving commodity.

The design effort focused on Nigeria, a country that had been developing its own national scale-up strategy and plan for chlorhexidine. This strategy identified the need to generate demand across caregivers, health care workers, and the private sector. Over the course of three months, a blended team including designers, donors, and implementing partners interviewed mothers, held community and professional workshops, shadowed birth attendants, and visited homes, antenatal clinics, and drug shops to understand the concerns informing decisions about umbilical cord care and to define the value proposition of chlorhexidine. Insights from these activities informed a broad range of design concepts. At each stage, the team solicited additional feedback on these concepts from the individuals, communities, and collaborators through rapid prototyping.

The outputs of this work were integrated into a demand generation toolkit. The toolkit includes recommendations, concepts, tools, and templates to be shared in Nigeria. The toolkit builds upon previous work to increase demand for chlorhexidine and other comparable products. The toolkit provides the Federal Ministries of Health, State Ministries of Health, partner organizations, and other groups with a starting point for thinking about the challenge and a head start on developing tools to address driving demand for chlorhexidine.

Design process

1. IMMERSION To establish a baseline understanding, the design team built on the national chlorhexidine scale-up strategy and implementation plan developed by the Ministry of Health and spoke with key stakeholders to understand Nigerian birth practices, the mothers' experience, the communities' context, and the role of different organizations in health behavior change. This input informed the creation of a map of the Nigerian birthing ecosystem and the design approach for the next phase.

2. RESEARCH To understand existing needs and behavior, the blended team visited communities and spoke with and observed mothers, families, birth attendants, chemists, community leaders, religious leaders, and antenatal clinic personnel. The team then synthesized their observations into insights about the barriers and opportunities in driving greater adoption and use of chlorhexidine.

3. CONCEPTING To translate these opportunities into initial concepts, the team held five participatory workshops with a wide range of stakeholders: four in Nigeria and one in New York. The participants in these sessions generated and prioritized concepts and constructed rapid prototypes of promising ideas. The team then took these ideas into communities to share them with people, gather feedback, and inspire new concepts directly with end-users and with both formal and informal health care providers in Nigeria.

4. STRATEGY The final concepts were integrated into a demand-generation toolkit with two parts: a guide, which provides details about the concepts and how they were developed, and an asset library, which provides images and editable templates. These resources offer a starting point for adapting these concepts across Nigeria and other countries to drive demand for this lifesaving product.

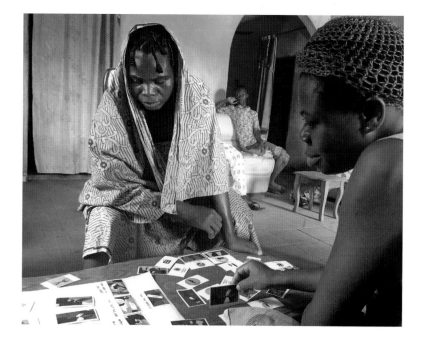

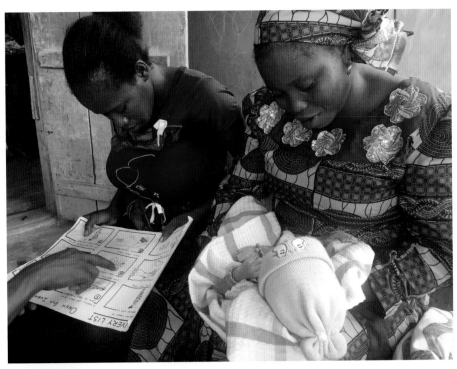

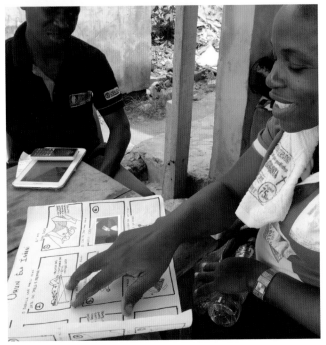

WORKSHOPS The project aimed to demonstrate the value of chlorhexidine to a range of stakeholders. A key factor was acknowledging and addressing other substances being used for umbilical cord care and the benefits yielded by switching to chlorhexidine. In a series of workshops, diverse stakeholders generated and prototyped concepts. These concepts were shared with community stakeholders in efforts to gather feedback and generate new concepts.

TOOLKIT A toolkit of resources (opposite) explains different approaches to driving demand and provides visual storytelling assets for communicating with stakeholders about the use of chlorhexidine. The assets are intended to be adapted for use in communities seeking to increase demand for chlorhexidine. To download the toolkit and learn about applying design thinking to global health, visit → www.usaid.gov/cii.

Assisted by birth attendant

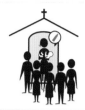

AWARENESS	PREPARATION	DELIVERY	POST-DELIVERY	SHARE

Jumoke heard about chlorhexidine at an orientation session a few months ago and has used it on four babies. During their first visit, Jumoke shares a flyer about chlorhexidine with Barifaa and they discuss the benefits. Jumoke mentions how chlorhexidine protects Barifaa a sample of the product.

At another visit, Jumoke shares a list of the products Barifaa will need for the delivery, including chlorhexidine. Barifaa says that she will need to space out her purchases based on her irregular income. She asks how much chlorhexidine costs. Jumoke says it costs about the same as rubbing alcohol maybe even cheaper since you only put it on once a day.

On the day of the delivery, Barifaa sends her oldest son to fetch Jumoke, who rushes to the home. Jumoke delivers the baby and cuts the cord with a blade, tying the end with a thread. She wipes the baby and puts chlorhexidine on the cord stump. She tells Barifaa not to wash the baby again until the next day. Jumoke announces the arrival of the baby to the village community.

Jumoke stops by each day to check on Barifaa and the baby. Barifaa is a little concerned that they waited a day before bathing the baby again and asks Jumoke if that might cause body odor issues. Jumoke reassures her that it will not and shares a message from their priest that babies who use chlorhexidine are especially blessed.

Once the naming ceremony has taken place, Barifaa and her husband bring the baby to church. Everyone remarks how beautiful the baby is and Barifaa credits Jumoke for all her help and advice, including her suggestion of chlorhexidine for the baby's cord.

OPPORTUNITIES

- Make birth attendants aware of chlorhexidine and how to use it.
- Develop materials to help communicate the value of chlorhexidine.

- Provide ways for birth attendants to share information and answer questions about chlorhexidine.

- Help attendants, mothers, and family members understand how to integrate chlorhexidine with other parts of the newborn care routine.

- Set expectations for how the cord will heal with use of chlorhexidine.

- Encourage mothers who have used chlorhexidine to share about the experience in their social circles.

CONCEPTS (DETAILS FOLLOW)

- Orientation and certificate
- Simple protection messaging

- Pictorial delivery list

- Pictorial routine

- Key community advocates

- Testimonials

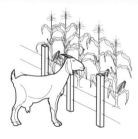

Fences protect crops from animals.

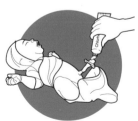

Chlorhexidine protects your baby's cord from infection.

Chlorhexidine 4% gel
Gentle and safe for your baby

Old Technology   **New Technology**

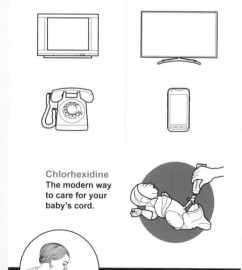

Chlorhexidine
The modern way to care for your baby's cord.

Chlorhexidine 4% gel
Gentle and safe for your baby

Emergency Department Signage

Graphic design is more than making beautiful logos and fancy letterheads. In health care, graphic design can improve outcomes and create better experiences for patients, staff, and clinicians. PearsonLloyd, a U.K.–based design firm, developed solutions to reduce violence and aggression in emergency departments of National Health Service (NHS) hospitals. More than 150 incidents of violence and aggression toward NHS hospital staff occur daily. The problem of violence costs the NHS system $90 million a year because of productivity loss, hiring of extra security, and staff absences.

Using in-depth ethnographic research, the design team discovered that the lack of clear information and guidance in EDs was a trigger for aggression. In this disorienting environment, patients felt frustrated by the slow pace of progression through the ED, and they perceived hospital staff to be inefficient because of long wait times.

PearsonLloyd designed visual graphics that improved signage and communication within the ED by representing the care journey. Consisting of graphic banners placed throughout the ED and a handheld printed map, this low-cost system helped patients feel oriented. Pilot testing showed impressive results. Threatening body language and aggressive behavior were reduced by 50%, and 75% of patients felt less frustration while waiting. Additionally, 88% of patients gained a clearer understanding of the ED process, and patient complaints about poor communication decreased by 57%.

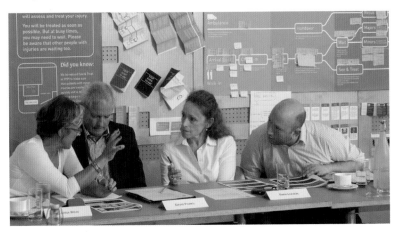

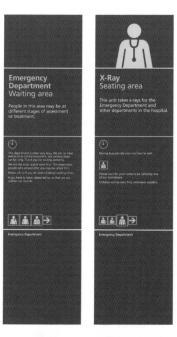

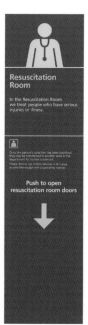

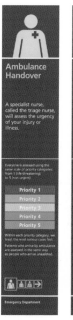

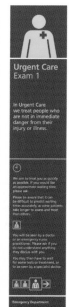

Arrivals

Please wait here to speak to a nurse. If you are a patient a nurse will assess your injuries or illness.

After this, please take a ticket for reception.

We aim to assess you within 15 minutes. Please be patient.

When the nurse has assessed your injury or illness, we will have a good idea of how serious it is and what type of treatment you may need. You then need to take a ticket to check in at reception, so your treatment can be prioritised. We aim to treat the most urgent injuries and illness first.

Emergency Department

Emergency Department
Waiting area

People in this area may be at different stages of assessment or treatment.

This department is often very busy. We aim to treat everyone as quickly as possible, but waiting times can be long. Thank you for waiting patiently.

We see the most urgent cases first. This means that people who arrived after you may be called first. Please ask us if you are worried about waiting times. If you have to leave, please tell us, so that we can update our records.

Emergency Department

X-Ray
Seating area

This unit takes x-rays for the Emergency Department and other departments in the hospital.

During busy periods you may have to wait.

Please wait for your name to be called by one of our technicians. Children will be seen first, whenever possible.

Emergency Department

Resuscitation Room

In the Resuscitation Room we treat people who have serious injuries or illness.

Once the patient's condition has been stabilised they may be transferred to another area in the department for further treatment. Please do not use mobile phones in this area, as sensitive equipment is operating nearby.

Push to open resuscitation room doors

Ambulance Handover

A specialist nurse, called the triage nurse, will assess the urgency of your injury or illness.

Everyone is assessed using the same scale of priority categories, from 1 (life-threatening) to 5 (non-urgent).

| Priority 1 |
| Priority 2 |
| Priority 3 |
| Priority 4 |
| Priority 5 |

Within each priority category, we treat the most serious cases first.

Patients who arrive by ambulance are assessed in the same way as people who arrive unassisted.

Emergency Department

Urgent Care
Exam 1

In Urgent Care we treat people who are not in immediate danger from their injury or illness.

We aim to treat you as quickly as possible. If you would like an approximate waiting time, please ask.

Please be aware that it can be difficult to predict waiting times accurately, as some patients take longer to assess and treat than others.

You will be seen by a doctor or an emergency nurse practitioner. Please ask if you do not understand anything they discuss with you.

You may then have to wait for some tests or treatment, or to be seen by a specialist doctor.

Emergency Department

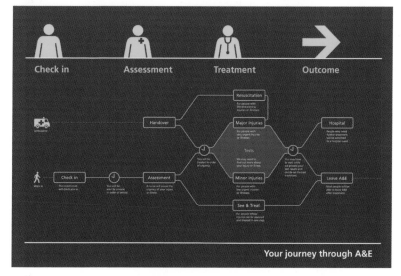

RESEARCH AND DEVELOPMENT (opposite) A team of designers and stakeholders studied the issues, challenges, and pain points of the ED process. They mapped the ideal patient journey through the ED, a document that served as a launching pad for generating solutions. Commissioned by the Design Council and funded by the Department of Health (UK). Signage © PearsonLloyd. Photo: Jack Cheatle

UNDERSTANDING THE ED (above) Information panels show patients their location and the exact stage of care in their ED journey. By looking at graphics posted throughout the ED, patients can understand why they are waiting and what factors will affect their wait times. They can anticipate what will happen during their next stage of care. The panels guide tired, suffering, and frightened patients through the chaos and confusion of a busy ED.

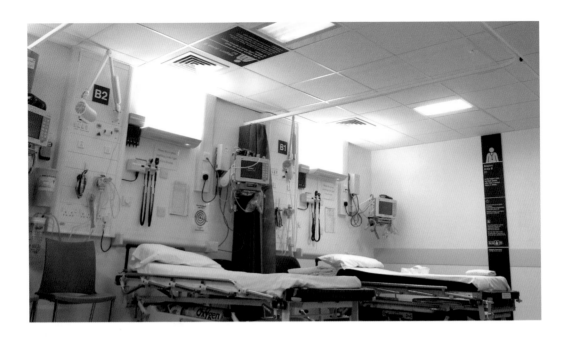

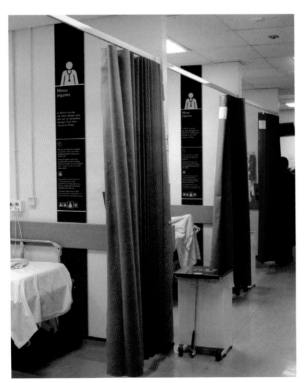

VERTICAL BANDS The information panels are designed as narrow vertical slices extending from floor to ceiling. The slices can be inserted into exam rooms, corridors, and waiting areas. In the resuscitation bay, a panel is fixed onto the ceiling. The design team recognized that a patient lying on a stretcher is more likely to be looking up at the ceiling than toward the side wall. This communication system represents a low-cost design solution that can be implemented in any ED. To date, sixteen hospitals in the U.K. have implemented the program, including Bristol Royal Infirmary, Belfast Health and Social Care Trust, and Royal London Hospital.

Project Collaborators: PearsonLloyd, Design Council, Department of Health, The Helyn Hamlyn Centre for Design, Tavistock Consulting, The Tavistock Institute, University of Bath

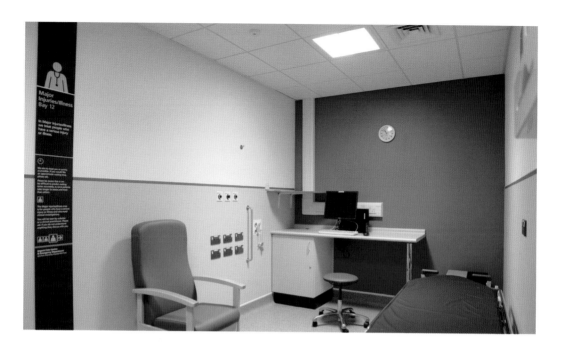

PROCESS MAP A paper leaflet given to patients supplements the signage in the ED. The leaflet shows a map of the four major stages of the patient journey: check-in, assessment, treatment, and outcome. A process map shows that each step has a purpose, and it addresses patients' frustration and uncertainty about why they are waiting. Photos © Simon Turner Photography and PearsonLloyd

READ MORE → designcouncil.org.uk/resources/ report/ae-design-challenge-impact-evaluation. → abetteraande.com/#solution → dezeen. com/2013/12/02/hospital-redesign-by-pearsonlloyd-reduces-violence-and-aggression/ → pearsonlloyd.com

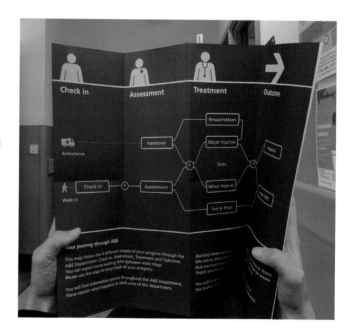

Exam Room

No one likes waiting rooms. You sit in an uncomfortable chair, skim old magazines, and watch tabloid talk shows or health advertisements on TV. Rarely do you get to see the doctor at the actual time of the appointment. At a typical visit to a clinic, most of the time is spent waiting, filling out forms, and interacting with nonphysician staff.

What if you could redesign the exam room from scratch? By studying doctor–patient interactions, the Center for Innovation at Mayo Clinic in Rochester, Minnesota, discovered that only 10–15% of the time is spent on the physical exam. This insight—combined with inspiration from the bathroom in the *Brady Bunch* TV show—led to the design of their Jack-and-Jill exam rooms. The *Brady Bunch* bathroom has two doors, and each door leads to a separate bedroom. Applied to exam rooms, this layout concept allows two consultation rooms to share an inner exam room, thereby saving square footage in the clinic.

As the new Dell Medical School at the University of Texas at Austin began planning for the launch of its specialty clinics, the school's embedded Design Institute for Health was asked to assist in the design of both the service model and the physical layout of the clinic. Instead of conforming to traditional designs, the team sought to reimagine the entire experience for people receiving and providing care. The clinics would disavow the fee-for-service model in lieu of a model of value-based, integrated care that moves the experience from a transactional to a relational focus.

Bold actions to empower the patient included eliminating the waiting room altogether. Upon entering the modern, spacious clinic, you check in with a concierge, who gives you an airport-like boarding pass with information about your assigned room. You proceed down a welcoming, hotel-like entryway to your care room, where you find prompts to make yourself comfortable; instructions on how to access free WiFi; a couch and chairs; a large, wall-mounted digital screen introducing you to your care team; and invitations to close the door and adjust the lights. At first glance, you see no exam table. In its place is a chair that converts into an examination table. The design layout equalizes the power balance by letting everyone in the room—patient, family members, clinicians—be at the same eye level.

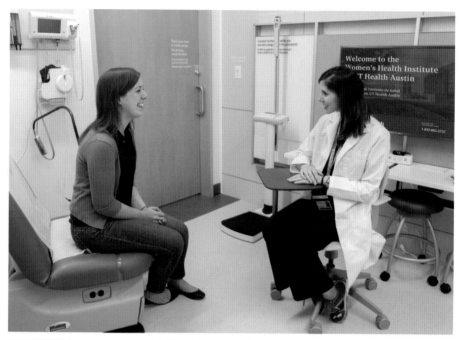

OWNERSHIP The care rooms are designed to be owned by the patients for the duration of their stay and to equalize the power balance between care team members and patients.

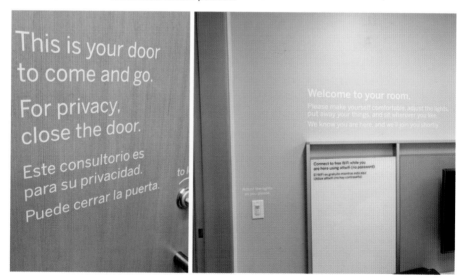

TALKING WALLS The room speaks directly to the patient, signaling a new kind of medical experience. Photos: Design Institute for Health, Dell Medical School

READ MORE → www.designinhealth.org/provoking-new-behaviors-ut-health-austin-clinic-experience-design/; → www.centerforinnovation.mayo.edu/jack-and-jill-rooms/

Labor and Delivery Unit

In the U.S., one third of babies are born by cesarean delivery; but up to 45% of these surgeries may not be medically indicated. The rates of cesarean delivery vary dramatically from hospital to hospital—from a modest 7% at some facilities to a whopping 70% at others. A study conducted by Ariadne Labs, a health system innovation center, and MASS Design Group, a nonprofit architecture firm, looked at how different aspects of the physical design of a hospital labor and delivery unit could lead to a higher rate of cesarean deliveries.

The team conducted a mixed-methods, descriptive study of a dozen hospitals and birth centers in the U.S. The study employs quantitative metrics—such as the distance between labor and delivery rooms (LDRs)—along with qualitative observations from team members. The size and shape of the labor and delivery unit, the standardization of patient rooms, and the distribution of nursing stations are design features that might influence the varying rates of cesarean deliveries among hospitals. Other metrics include the ratio of operating rooms (ORs) to LDRs and the distances between rooms. A shortage of LDRs, easy access to ORs, or the need to walk long distances in a jumbo-sized facility could spur clinicians to move patients more quickly through labor and delivery, yielding more cesarean deliveries. For these reasons, the health care facility in which a woman chooses to give birth is a strong predictor for a cesarean delivery.

In addition to researching a specific outcome (higher cesarian rates), the study illuminates the broader effects of hospital layout on morale and productivity. For example, when a hospital changed its nursing stations from a larger, collaborative space to smaller, dispersed spaces closer to LDRs, nurses reported feeling isolated and depressed. Thus, a well-intentioned design change yielded an unexpected side effect. Summarized and excerpted here are elements of this remarkable study, which demonstrates the power of methodical design research to yield rich insights about human behavior and the built environment. By combining evidence-based design with improvements to design processes, we hope to provide helpful guidance to clinician–architect collaborators who intend to build environments that support better care at lower cost.

DISTANCE FROM NURSING STATION TO LDR

The average distances between different rooms within a health care unit contribute to staff workload. The nursing station is a central hub of activity on a labor and delivery unit. Many hospitals even refer to these locations as "control centers." Sometimes they are used by physicians, midwives, and students as well as by nursing staff.

Distances between nursing stations and LDRs vary widely, from an average distance of 23 feet at Sharp Mary Birch Hospital for Women & Newborns, where nurses sit just steps away from each of the four rooms in their pod, to an average distance of 114 feet at football-field-sized University Medical Center of Princeton at Plainsboro, where nurses and physicians reported frequently having to run from room to room to care for patients. We found that longer average distances between the nursing station and LDRs may be associated with higher cesarean rates.

As units grow in size, some hospitals employ a distributed nursing station model, in which smaller substations are located throughout the unit to increase patient access to nurses. We heard from facilities that this model may have the unintended consequence of disrupting clinician/nurse communication. Beth Israel Deaconess Medical Center has found that close proximity of LDRs to small, distributed nursing stations threatens patient confidentiality: "I worry about patient privacy. You don't have any place to go to have a private or difficult conversation. Those things end up happening in the kitchen or med room."

Despite proximity of LDRs to the nursing station at Tuba City Regional Health Care Corporation, the unit layout hinders efficient patient care. "If you want something, you have to either search for it or walk to the other end of the unit" (Acting Supervisor). The unit hasn't been significantly renovated since it was designed for a labor > delivery > recovery > postpartum model of care.

"We find ourselves using the old patient rooms because of their proximity to the nursing station, even though they're dingier. You're in and out so much, that you need to be close."—Director, Women's Services, Merit Health Natchez

Since moving to the new unit, nurses at The Mother Baby Center have struggled to adjust to the larger floor area and distances from their colleagues.

Average distance from the nurse station to the LDR
Measured variation within facility study set

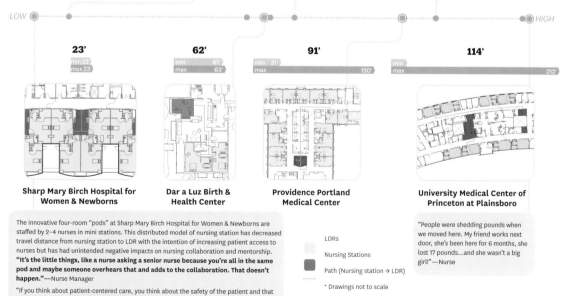

LOW ● ● ● ● ● ● HIGH

23'
min 22'
max 23'

62'
min 61'
max 63'

91'
min 31'
max 150'

114'
min
max 212'

Sharp Mary Birch Hospital for Women & Newborns

Dar a Luz Birth & Health Center

Providence Portland Medical Center

University Medical Center of Princeton at Plainsboro

The innovative four-room "pods" at Sharp Mary Birch Hospital for Women & Newborns are staffed by 2–4 nurses in mini stations. This distributed model of nursing station has decreased travel distance from nursing station to LDR with the intention of increasing patient access to nurses but has had unintended negative impacts on nursing collaboration and mentorship. **"It's the little things, like a nurse asking a senior nurse because you're all in the same pod and maybe someone overhears that and adds to the collaboration. That doesn't happen."**—Nurse Manager

"If you think about patient-centered care, you think about the safety of the patient and that takes a team. Yes, the nurse is very available. Can they be there in 10 seconds versus thirty? Sure. But...It's not just about distance."—Nurse Manager

☐ LDRs

☐ Nursing Stations

▨ Path (Nursing station → LDR)

* Drawings not to scale

"People were shedding pounds when we moved here. My friend works next door, she's been here for 6 months, she lost 17 pounds...and she wasn't a big girl!"—Nurse

TOO MANY OPERATING ROOMS? The ratios among different types of dedicated space within health care facilities can influence clinical outcomes. There may be a correlation between higher ratios of ORs to LDRs and higher cesarean rates. OR access is a critical component of capacity for performing both scheduled and emergent cesarean deliveries. Access is a function of the physical space (number and availability of rooms) and of access to staff to provide anesthesia and perform the surgery. This study measured OR access as a ratio of ORs to LDRs for each facility. The study sought to find out how the relative capacity of the unit to perform a cesarean delivery as opposed to a vaginal delivery would affect treatment intensity. Based on insights from a facilities manager on the research team's

advisory board, the team hypothesized that a higher ratio of ORs to LDRs may be associated with higher cesarean rates because of a "supply-induced demand mechanism": the more readily accessible the OR, the fewer the barriers to performing surgery. Of note is that freestanding birth centers do not contain ORs—patients who require cesarean delivery must be transported to the nearest hospital.

The number of ORs on a labor and delivery unit depends on several factors. First, units serving higher acuity patient populations, which are more likely to need cesarean deliveries, require greater OR access. Greater socioeconomic context, such as the percentage of patients covered by Medicaid, may better elucidate the role of design in sustaining or alleviating disparities in care.

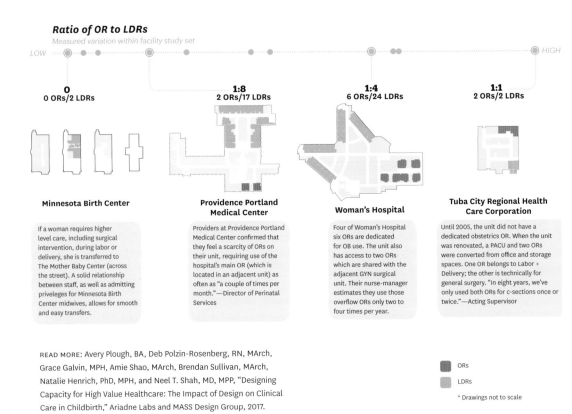

Ratio of OR to LDRs
Measured variation within facility study set

LOW .... HIGH

0
0 ORs/2 LDRs

1:8
2 ORs/17 LDRs

1:4
6 ORs/24 LDRs

1:1
2 ORs/2 LDRs

Minnesota Birth Center

If a woman requires higher level care, including surgical intervention, during labor or delivery, she is transferred to The Mother Baby Center (across the street). A solid relationship between staff, as well as admitting privileges for Minnesota Birth Center midwives, allows for smooth and easy transfers.

Providence Portland Medical Center

Providers at Providence Portland Medical Center confirmed that they feel a scarcity of ORs on their unit, requiring use of the hospital's main OR (which is located in an adjacent unit) as often as "a couple of times per month."—Director of Perinatal Services

Woman's Hospital

Four of Woman's Hospital six ORs are dedicated for OB use. The unit also has access to two ORs which are shared with the adjacent GYN surgical unit. Their nurse-manager estimates they use those overflow ORs only two to four times per year.

Tuba City Regional Health Care Corporation

Until 2005, the unit did not have a dedicated obstetrics OR. When the unit was renovated, a PACU and two ORs were converted from office and storage spaces. One OR belongs to Labor + Delivery; the other is technically for general surgery. "In eight years, we've only used both ORs for c-sections once or twice."—Acting Supervisor

READ MORE: Avery Plough, BA, Deb Polzin-Rosenberg, RN, MArch, Grace Galvin, MPH, Amie Shao, MArch, Brendan Sullivan, MArch, Natalie Henrich, PhD, MPH, and Neel T. Shah, MD, MPP, "Designing Capacity for High Value Healthcare: The Impact of Design on Clinical Care in Childbirth," Ariadne Labs and MASS Design Group, 2017.

ORs

LDRs

* Drawings not to scale

MAXIMUM DISTANCE BETWEEN LDRS For staff caring for multiple patients in a single shift, the distance between LDRs can have a strong impact on workload. Closely spaced, efficiently laid-out units contrast with vast, sprawling units, where nurses may find themselves literally running between rooms. During a site visit, one obstetrician said he had invested in gels for his shoes after the move to the new unit: "The path going from room to room to go to a supply room, it really kills our staffing."

Larger rooms are needed to accommodate laboring and the procedural aspect of the delivery itself, and for the expanded staff that accompanies the presence of a second patient (the infant) and for specialists in case of an emergency. Therefore, large patient room size is a unique labor and delivery design challenge that can be dealt with in ways that are more and less efficient. Sharp Mary Birch Hospital for Women & Newborns has clustered its 22 rooms in such a way as to maximize efficiency and compactness between sets of rooms, although this hospital's absolute maximum distance is the highest in our research sample. In contrast, University Medical Center of Princeton at Plainsboro, which contends with the next highest distances between LDRS, has only eight rooms, but the rooms are lined up along the periphery of a long, curving corridor—probably the least efficient arrangement.

MOST EFFICIENT LAYOUT

LEAST EFFICIENT LAYOUT

Sharp Mary Birch Hospital for Women & Newborns Hospital
Distance between four rooms
13'

University Medical Center of Princeton at Plainsboro
Distance between four rooms
119'

Maximum distance between LDRs
Measured variation within facilitystudy set

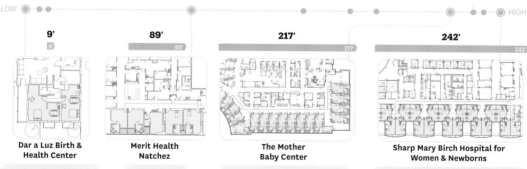

LOW ── HIGH

9'

89'

217'

242'

Dar a Luz Birth & Health Center

At Dar a Luz, the two birth suites are just steps from one another. In the case that both rooms are occupied by patients, midwives can easily move between rooms to monitor labors.

Merit Health Natchez

"It's easy to move around the unit."
—Director, Women's Services

The Mother Baby Center

The Mother Baby Center complained that building codes required spacious LDRs, which necessarily increased travel distance between rooms. One physician acknowledged the tipping point at which a single-floor unit design becomes impractical (versus distributing the unit among several stacked floors)—"otherwise you end up with the football field situation, taking forever to get from one place to another."—Obstetrician

Sharp Mary Birch Hospital for Women & Newborns

Because of the four-room pod layout at Sharp Mary Birch, the maximum distance between rooms is effectively 13' for floor nurses. Charge nurses and providers must still contend with the greater travel distance in carrying out their daily work. The pod structure also impedes distribution of workload, as nurses rely on only those 1 or 2 other nurses working in their individual pod to cover their patients for a break, for example. "The culture is so ingrained to be in a pod, that no one wants to leave the pod. We don't get our breaks."—Nurse Manager

COLLABORATIVE SPACES Oportunities to share knowledge and to communicate with colleagues are critical to a sense of team accountability. We analyzed the ratio of staff areas designed for collaborative interaction among team members to the total staff area. The team predicted that collaborative spaces would lead to a greater sense of accountability for providing optimal care and would drive treatment intensity down.

The Mother Baby Center has a high proportion of collaborative staff spaces (nearly all), while Woman's Hospital has very few collaborative spaces—staff work and take breaks as groups of nurses or clinicians, excluding the rest of the team. Beth Israel Deaconess Medical Center and Tuba City Regional Health Care Corporation Regional both have centrally located common work areas. At Providence Portland Medical Center, inclusive team huddles happen in the hall outside a snack room near the nursing station.

At University of Chicago Medical Center, the "Board Room" is for physicians and midwives; nurses enter this room only to give reports. Commonly, hospital unit break rooms are divided among staff as well. At Tuba City Regional Health Care Corporation, the space designated "Common Lounge" is, in practice, only for nurses, though it is rarely used because of its distance from the nursing station. (Instead, nurses perch on a trash can lid in the patient kitchen to grab a snack.)

A relative lack of collaborative staff areas may contribute to higher cesarean rates. Our contextual findings further clarify, however, that increased accountability does not automatically translate into higher or lower cesarean rates. Team culture and overall intentions must be understood. In tertiary settings, increased accountability may actually increase cesarean rates as patients are monitored more closely.

"Of course, it makes sense to have everyone working in the same area. I don't know how we're going to achieve more of that in the new space. Ideally, it would be great to have nursing in the room as well."
—Medical Director, Women's Services, University of Chicago Medical Center

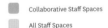
Collaborative Staff Spaces
All Staff Spaces

Ratio of total staff area to collaborative staff area
Measured variation within facility study set

LOW   HIGH

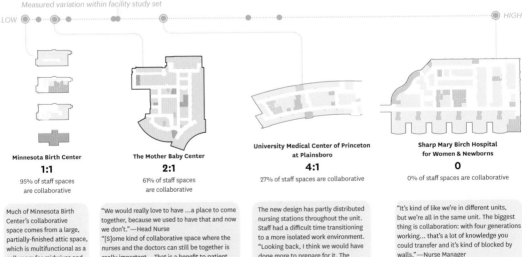

Minnesota Birth Center
1:1
95% of staff spaces are collaborative

The Mother Baby Center
2:1
61% of staff spaces are collaborative

University Medical Center of Princeton at Plainsboro
4:1
27% of staff spaces are collaborative

Sharp Mary Birch Hospital for Women & Newborns
0
0% of staff spaces are collaborative

Much of Minnesota Birth Center's collaborative space comes from a large, partially-finished attic space, which is multifunctional as a call-room for midwives and a collaborative work space for all staff.

"We would really love to have ...a place to come together, because we used to have that and now we don't."—Head Nurse
"[S]ome kind of collaborative space where the nurses and the doctors can still be together is really important... That is a benefit to patient care. In this building we have the nurse's lounge and the doctor's lounge. So we find ourselves— or I do, often—sitting and having my dinner in the nurses lounge...that team aspect of things is very important in the care of patients."
—Obstetrician

The new design has partly distributed nursing stations throughout the unit. Staff had a difficult time transitioning to a more isolated work environment. "Looking back, I think we would have done more to prepare for it. The social aspects...everyone used to be together. We are so spread out that some people were really depressed." —Director, Patient Care Services

"It's kind of like we're in different units, but we're all in the same unit. The biggest thing is collaboration: with four generations working... that's a lot of knowledge you could transfer and it's kind of blocked by walls."—Nurse Manager

ROOM STANDARDIZATION Another design feature that contributes to staff workload is the degree of standardization among patient rooms. Health care design experts frequently argue that standardizing the headwall location in patient rooms improves staff efficiency by reducing the cognitive effort required to reorient to a unique layout within each room. In theory, when rooms are standardized, a nurse or clinician can enter any room on the unit and know immediately where to find necessary tools, instead of having to expend mental energy recalling the setup within a particular room. Based on this theory, we predicted that room standardization might decrease workload.

In our facility sample, the team observed varying degrees of LDR standardization: from completely unique room layouts (more common among birth centers), to standardized but mirrored layouts (same headwall layout located on different sides in different rooms), to same-handed rooms (with headwalls located on the same side in each room). Our sample as a whole was evenly distributed among these three degrees of LDR standardization, but birth centers were uniformly nonstandardized. Typically, birth centers are in renovated houses or offices, where existing building conditions limit the options for standardization within labor and delivery rooms. Natchez was an outlier among the hospitals we studied—its five LDRs had fairly unique room layouts, resulting from a history of selective renovations to the unit.

Although it's commonly believed within the field of health care architecture that standardization improves efficiency, there is little evidence to support this claim. Furthermore, the construction requirements for achieving same-handed rooms are significant and costly—adjacent rooms must each be afforded a separate chase for plumbing and medical gases rather than sharing a common chase; this course of action significantly increases the cost of construction for these facilities. Staff at University Medical Center of Princeton at Plainsboro indicated that same-handedness had actually negatively affected efficiency—the additional chases required even larger LDRs, which create a workload burden by further increasing the distances between rooms.

Room standardization

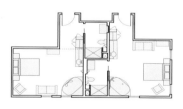

LOW

*Each room has
unique layout*

**Minnesota
Birth Center**

Typically, birth centers like Minnesota Birth Center occupy renovated houses or offices, where existing building conditions limit the options for standardization within labor and delivery rooms.

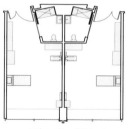

MEDIUM

*Standardized room setup but
mirrored back to back.*

**University of Chicago
Medical Center**

Despite the commonly-held belief that standardization improves efficiency, there is little evidence to support the claim that same-handed rooms increase patient safety or staff efficiency over mirrored rooms, like this one.

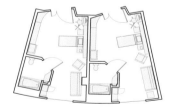

HIGH

*Same-handed rooms in which
headwalls are located on the same
side of each room.*

**The Mother
Baby Center**

Staff at University Medical Center of Princeton at Plainsboro indicated that same-handedness had actually negatively impacted efficiency—the additional chases required even larger LDRs, which further increased the distances between adjacent rooms.

Cholera Treatment Center

The first clinical report of cholera came ten months after the devastating earthquake hit Haiti in 2010. The disease spread across the country and soon became one of the largest and deadliest cholera epidemics in recent history, with a death toll of nearly 10,000. Like hundreds of health care facilities across the country, Les Centres GHESKIO quickly deployed cholera treatment tents, intended as a short-term response. But as the epidemic continued, the tents became the permanent mainstays for cholera treatment, despite being hot, uncomfortable, and undignifying.

Cholera is an acute diarrheal disease that is spread through fecal contamination of food and water. Although cholera in its most severe form can cause death from dehydration within hours, it is a wholly preventable and treatable disease. Haiti's infrastructure was hindering the nation's ability to adequately respond to the outbreak.

Dr. Jean William Pape, founder and executive director of GHESKIO, asked MASS Design Group to help create a permanent cholera center. His request was simple and revolutionary: Could the center address Haiti's systemic infrastructural shortfallings and treat patients with dignity? MASS designed the Cholera Treatment Center (CTC) to break the cycle of cholera by treating sick patients in dignifying spaces, increasing staff comfort and efficiency, and responding to systemic challenges using local water and sanitation infrastructure.

Designed to treat 100 patients at a time, the layout optimizes staff and patient flow. Patients entering the facility are greeted by staff, who invite them to shower and change into a hospital gown in a private room. Nurses oversee patients from a centralized station. To simplify routine sterilization, pour-flush stations are distributed throughout the building, reducing the distance staff need to travel to dispose of buckets of waste. All building materials—including metal screens, stucco walls, concrete floors, and custom-fabricated beds—were chosen for their durability, their infection-resistant properties, and/or their ability to withstand extensive washing with chlorine.

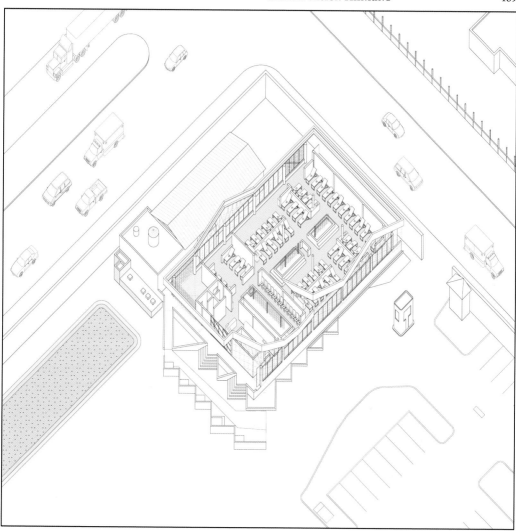

WATER COLLECTION SYSTEM Rainwater collected along the center of the roof is channeled to the northwest edge, where it drains into a tank built into a planter inside the CTC.

CISTERN The water collected from the roof and stored in the tank is pumped to a rooftop tank on an adjacent building for storage, filtering, and reuse.

ORAL REHYDRATION SOLUTION Filtered rainwater is piped back to the CTC, where it is mixed with salts to act as a rapid rehydration tool for patients.

ANAEROBIC BAFFLED REACTOR Wastewater is piped into a 4-chambered reactor, where the waste is broken down into biomass sludge and fertigation water to be used on-site.

LEACHING FIELD Treated wastewater is irrigated into a leaching field, where it soaks into the ground. Further impurities are removed by plant life.

The facility prioritizes the comfort and dignity of its users. An expansive ceiling; a perforated screen facade; and large, slow-revolution, high-volume fans bring in fresh air and cool the space through stack effect, cross ventilation, and low-energy design strategies. Interior vegetation makes efficient use of rainwater runoff while bringing natural beauty indoors. Half-height walls and trellis screens provide privacy between patients. The plantings also provide emotional respite and contribute to improved patient outcomes.

The design responds to the local site and systemic conditions by providing an off-the-grid water and sanitation infrastructure. The roof, which is designed to help bring in natural daylight, also collects rainwater, which is stored in underground cisterns, treated, and then used in showers and sinks. The facility decontaminates waste on-site using a leaching field combined with anaerobic baffled reactor technology. The system is designed to achieve 99.99% removal and inactivation of *cholera vibrio* and other pathogenic organisms. The CTC has the capacity to treat more than 250,000 gallons of sewage a year, thereby helping reduce water table contamination.

The CTC is designed to maximize its impact over the long term—not only through the quality performance of the facility but also through capacity building and economic investment opportunities during the construction process. The building's metal screen facades were designed using a high-tech digital design process to optimize light, ventilation, and privacy based on programmatic needs. The design was implemented through partnerships with Haitian craftsmen. Led by local artisans, the team developed a custom folding strategy that offered precision and highlighted the human handprint involved in creating the project: over 8,000 apertures were cut and bent by hand. The beds, chairs, and cabinetry were designed in partnership with international experts and manufactured locally, largely on-site. Along with additional architectural and construction-training workshops onsite, this collaborative, craft-based approach became a means to promote safer, more effective building practices and to invest in the educational and economic growth of the community.

The Cholera Treatment Center models more than a user-driven health care environment; it offers an example of an entirely different approach to post-disaster development. The center treats acute patient need while investing in local economic development and addressing the environmental conditions that contributed to the cholera outbreak.

Strategies for patient comfort and dignity

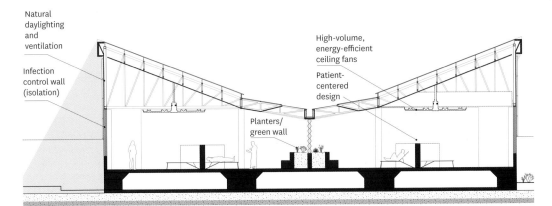

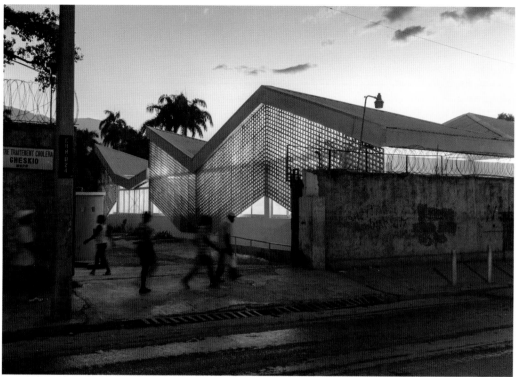

© Iwan Baan

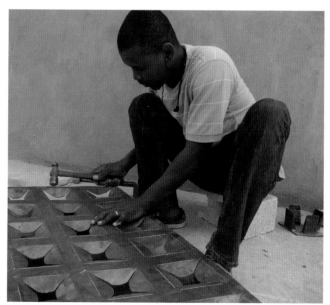

"*Architecture and health are inseparable. A building that is ugly, with no fresh air, no dignity or common sense, is a place people will avoid, and this encourages epidemics.*"

DR. JEAN WILLIAM PAPE

GHESKIO CHOLERA TREATMENT CENTER Design: MASS Design Group. Location: Port-au-Prince, Haiti. Building Area: 695 square meters. Capacity: 100 beds. Opened: 2015. Partners: Fall Creek Engineering, Mazzetti, Virginia Tech Center for Design Research

Sensory Arts Garden

The Sensory Arts Garden at The Els Center of Excellence in Jupiter, Florida, is a therapeutic environment serving individuals on the autism spectrum. The garden's program, design, and construction involved a close collaboration between landscape architect David Kamp and the Els Center's Director of Programs, Marlene Sotelo, and its Occupational Therapy Consultant, Amy Wagenfeld. With the Sensory Arts Garden, the Center expands its therapeutic program into a vibrant outdoor setting, thereby welcoming nature as an essential partner in health and wellness.

Serenity, security, and restoration are the foundation of a design that honors individual strengths and preferences, addresses the realities of sensory regulation challenges common to individuals on the spectrum, and welcomes all garden visitors from the Els community and beyond. By embracing the many facets of a complex disorder, the garden demonstrates that a nurturing sensory environment is a dynamic tool that supports individuals with autism in achieving their full capacities.

At every scale—from overall configuration, to material selection, to the subtlest of design details—the garden reflects a carefully researched and nuanced response to the breadth and complexity of autism. Considerations for routine, pattern, repetition, and wayfinding informed the overall site design; at the same time, a degree of openness and flexibility allows all visitors to experience continued discovery, free play, and autonomy.

Every material and furnishing was considered for its appropriateness, safety, and therapeutic potential. At key moments, changes in color or texture of the ground plane—such as from smoothly paved to roughly pebbled—signal changes in sensory experience or activity and draw one's focus toward the body and the senses. The garden is designed to honor individual strengths and preferences, reduce stress and anxiety, encourage social interaction and exploration, and, most important, welcome and engage all, regardless of age, ability, or preference. This inclusive design was achieved through a balance of clear circulation and form and a diversity of sensory experiences.

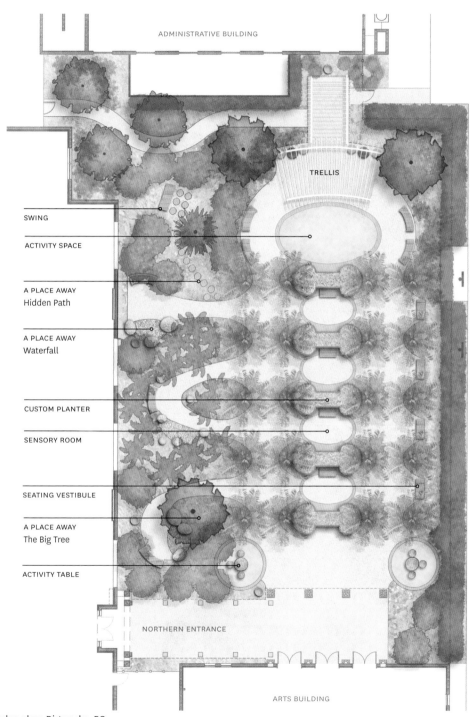

ADMINISTRATIVE BUILDING

TRELLIS

SWING

ACTIVITY SPACE

A PLACE AWAY
Hidden Path

A PLACE AWAY
Waterfall

CUSTOM PLANTER

SENSORY ROOM

SEATING VESTIBULE

A PLACE AWAY
The Big Tree

ACTIVITY TABLE

NORTHERN ENTRANCE

ARTS BUILDING

Garden plan: Dirtworks, PC

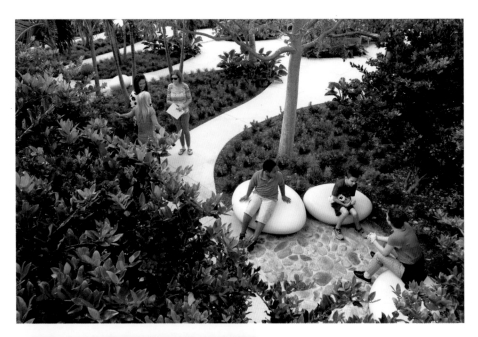

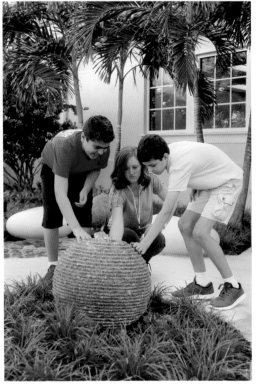

SENSORY SPACES Reduced and integrated sensory spaces provide a calming counterpoint for an individual who may experience hypersensitivity or seek a moment of respite or refuge. Each space features a seating area for individual or group use. Tactile engagement and gross motor skills are enhanced through interaction with the pebble paving.

WATER SPHERES Low to the ground and tucked into planting beds, water spheres provide opportunities for many sensory experiences, including the proprioceptive and vestibular. Their placement requires visitors to squat, reach, and balance. Smooth and rigid spheres offer varied tactile engagement.

FOCUSED SPACE Standing or sitting within a ring can help an autistic individual become less agitated. This circular personal space encourages focused attention and supports discussions among therapists, teachers, and students. Here, the muted color palette of the plantings enhances feelings of serenity and tranquility.

VARIED EXPERIENCES The garden's seemingly simple layout accommodates a variety of needs: solitude and socialization, respite and activity, focused engagement or therapy, and simple distractions. A range of seating types throughout the garden provides varying levels of proprioceptive and vestibular experiences.

Photos: Robin Hill

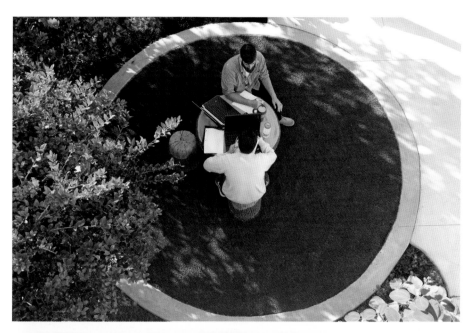

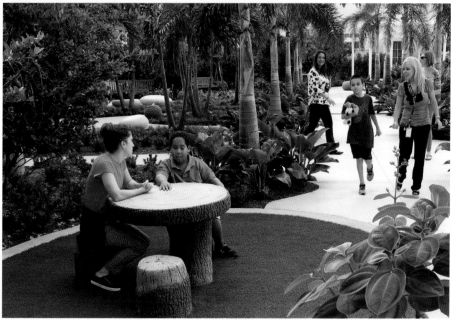

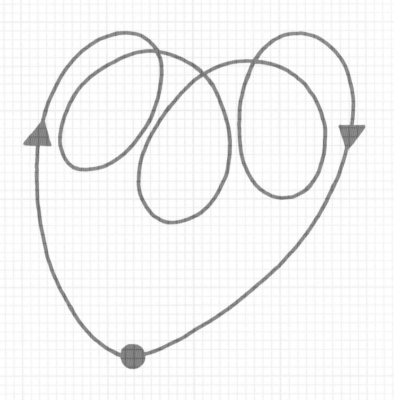

Learn more. This book is just the beginning. It's a handbook and a primer to get you started on your own journey of human-centered research and creative invention. There is so much more to read, do, and make. We end this book with suggestions for creating a health design lab at your school or university and for generating new design challenges and coursework. You will also find more design principles and resources for further study. Often, people don't pay attention to how a service or product is designed until it stops working. Health design problems are all around us—on every street, in every city, in every clinic and hospital.

Health Design Lab

When we think of creative spaces, the images that come to mind may be an artist's studio or an architecture office—not a hospital. But creative spaces are as important to health care as they are to artists and designers. Creative spaces help to encourage making, build collaboration within teams, and inspire us to think differently.

Alas, the physical spaces found in health care settings rarely inspire creativity. Nursing and medical students sit for hours in fixed chairs in theater-style lecture halls. Physicians, when not seeing patients, sit alone in front of computers in their offices. Administrators go from meeting to meeting in conference rooms furnished with long tables and large screens displaying dull presentations.

Working in a creative space can snap people out of their routines by enabling new modes of thought and promoting conversation. Think of a Health Design Lab as a gym where clinicians, nurses, and administrators can exercise their creative muscles.

The Health Design Lab at Thomas Jefferson University blends scientific and artistic creativity. The Lab was inspired by design studios, maker spaces, and biomedical research labs. Medical, nursing, and other health science students use the Lab to build prototypes of new medical devices, brainstorm better solutions in health care delivery, and create 3D-printed anatomical models for surgical planning.

The Lab's flexible environment and 24/7 open access enable teams to co-create at any time. Patients, clinicians, researchers, nurses, and administrators take advantage of whiteboards, sticky notes, Sharpies, and moveable worktables on wheels to ideate and make. They work together in teams to understand the complex problems in health care and develop ideas and solutions. The Lab acts as an innovation garage that encourages users to make, tinker, and test. Teams use the Lab to build low-resolution prototypes of new medical products using materials like foamcore, cardboard, and Legos. 3D printers, micro-electronics, design software, and other fabrication tools allow teams to build higher-resolution prototypes. The Lab is a safe space for experimentation—it grants permission to do, test, fail, and try again.

Building a Health Design Lab

Embed the Lab within a hospital or clinic. Make accessing it easy for clinicians, nurses, and patients.

Choose furniture that is easy to move around. Put wheels on everything.

Prioritize low-resolution prototyping. Most people don't know how to use a 3D printer or a laser cutter, but anyone can tinker with everyday materials.

Provide whiteboards to encourage people to draw, diagram, and doodle.

Make the space organic. Trying changing the layout every few months.

Allow teams to display their work on walls and on project visualization boards.

Workshops for clinical teams may require minimal software and supplies. An incubator program for developing medical products will require more sophisticated resources.

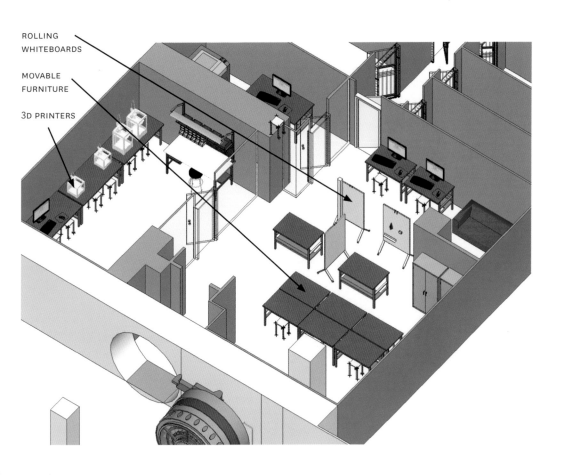

ROLLING
WHITEBOARDS

MOVABLE
FURNITURE

3D PRINTERS

PROTOYPING CART Colorful supplies allow people to think with their hands, inviting them to play and imagine. The prototyping cart contains tools and materials for running a design workshop, a brainstorming session, or a making activity. If you need to carry supplies to another location, use a plastic box or suitcase to house prototyping supplies and keep them organized.

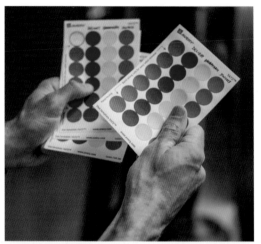

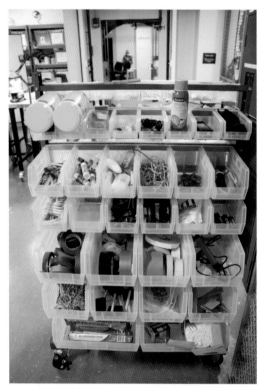

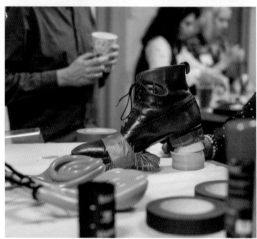

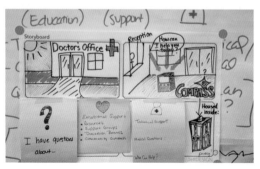

PROTOTYPING SUPPLIES

Markers and pens
Sticky notes
Pipe cleaners
Popsicle sticks
Scrap paper
Tin foil
Modeling clay
Painter's tape
Clear tape
Glue sticks
Rubber bands

Zip ties
Yarn
Hot glue gun
Paper clips/staples/tacks
Scissors/blades
Assortment of cheap toys
Cardboard
Dot stickers
Legos
Rulers
Foam sheets

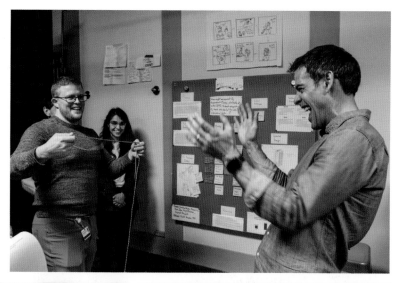

WORK IN PROGRESS
Students and faculty gather often to debrief. Each team displays its research, ideas, and prototypes on a dedicated project visualization board.

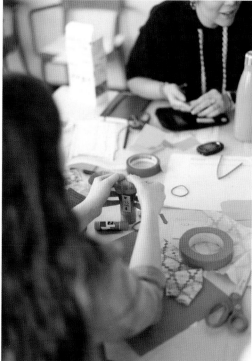

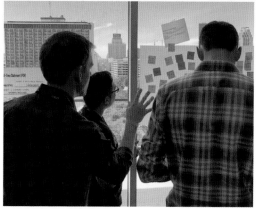

ACTIVE LEARNING Working with physical materials is concrete and inspiring. Photo: David Campbell

HACK YOUR OWN CREATIVE SPACE Don't worry if you lack the resources or space to build a permanent Health Design Lab. Improvise to convert any room into a creative environment. One of our favorite workarounds is converting the walls and windows in an ordinary conference room into temporary whiteboards. Cover surfaces with large sticky pads (25 x 30 inches) or rolls of white paper. Rearrange furniture to allow teams to claim an area as their own pop-up design studio. Fill a table with materials like markers, sticky notes, scissors, tape, and cardboard for sketching and storyboarding. Encourage physical making by bringing in prototyping supplies like glue guns, scrap paper, modeling clay, and tin foil. Simple interventions like these can change traditional meetings into participatory events where teams think and behave creatively.

Medical Futures Lab

The Medical Futures Lab at Rice University aims to improve the patient experience through human-centered approaches to technology in medicine. Led by a humanities-trained researcher, Kirsten Ostherr, PhD, MPH, the Lab brings together clinicians from the nearby medical center to work with university students and faculty from engineering, visual arts, business, social sciences, and architecture. The Lab has a unique focus on undergraduate (baccalaureate) learners. In the Lab, premedical undergraduate students learn how to solve complex, real-world, patient-centered problems involving communication and visualization of information in health care.

Following a process of human-centered design supported by readings in media theory, information and communication technology research, digital health case studies, and health policy reports, teams of students collaborate with clinician "problem owners" to create solutions. Lab leaders work with clinicians in advance to clearly define the problem scope. Clinicians and other faculty mentors provide guidance, technical training, access to relevant environments for observation, key people to interview, and feedback on design prototypes. Projects have resulted in short videos, communication scripts, graphic design, virtual 3D models, infographics, game design, text-messaging campaigns, and app development.

The Medical Futures Lab is part of a Medical Humanities program that is populated largely by premed STEM majors who want to explore the human side of caring for patients. Students internalize the human dimensions of doctoring through this kind of creative, team-based, hands-on work. By engaging in health design thinking, premedical students learn to appreciate the importance of developing empathy by listening, becoming attuned to storytelling, and understanding the lived contexts in which patients experience health and illness. These are core objectives of the growing movement in Health Humanities for premedical and medical students worldwide. The experience of the students at the Medical Futures Lab has shown that health design thinking is a highly effective method for teaching these values. Such training helps future doctors cultivate the skills to lead this kind of work in their clinical careers.

HUMANITIES-BASED APPROACH The Lab has developed humanities-based design techniques tailored to address their special focus on communication and visualization. Some of these practices tap the power of metaphors, similes, and other analogies as creative thinking and prototyping tools. Through these exercises, students explore emotional, contextual, aesthetic, and narrative aspects of problems that might be invisible when seen through a narrow biomedical view of health and disease.

For example, many of the barriers that patients face involve nonmedical aspects of their lives, such as financial pressures from poverty and high medical bills, stress from pervasive structural racism, confusion and intimidation from medical jargon, or fatigue from being a caregiver of a chronically ill patient. What tools do these people already turn to in their lives to help them stay organized or connected, or to find temporary escape from daily stresses? What do they find helpful or pleasurable about using some websites or apps that keeps them coming back? What compelling stories or images engage their interest? The Lab uses analogy exercises to ask: How might a team's design solution be like those other experiences that effectively engage their users?

The teams use storyboards as tools for discovery, synthesis, and usability testing. Principles from cinematic narrative are employed to show how a story takes place through a cause–effect chain that is often nonlinear and recursive. This framing helps students think through the constraints and opportunities involved in their solution. For example, if a mobile app is meant to connect a surgical patient through the continuum of care, from pre-op to post-op to discharge, the patient must not only have a device that can run the app but must also download the app, be motivated to install it, log in, and use it, and then—most important—the patient must experience an incentive to return to the app to enter the status updates that the team expects will help solve their problem.

Storyboarding helps address a common mistake in digital health design: the assumption that once a tool becomes available, people will automatically use it, exactly as intended. The Lab addresses this fallacy by assigning a team member the role of devil's advocate, who questions every encounter the user has with the design solution. These advocates can add frames to the storyboard to map out spaces where the process could go awry, prompting the team to refine their prototype.

Defining a design challenge

A well-defined design challenge is specific enough that a student team of nonexperts can develop a viable solution that will truly benefit patients, caregivers, and/or health professionals. The problem must also be challenging enough to merit fifteen weeks of dedicated effort and account for the genuine complexity of the U.S. health care system. The Medical Futures Lab at Rice University has addressed problems such as . . .

Sepsis awareness for home caregivers

Patient enrollment in clinical trials for personalized cancer drug therapies

End-of-life preferences for pediatric cystic fibrosis patients

Goal-setting communication between doctors and patients with type 1 diabetes

Team communication on cardiovascular intensive care unit rounds

READ MORE Kirsten Ostherr, "Digital Humanities and Design Thinking," in Nathan Carlin *et al.*, eds., *Teaching Health Humanities* (New York: Oxford University Press, 2019); Kirsten Ostherr, ed., *Applied Media Studies* (New York: Routledge, 2018).

Health Design Curriculum

Health design thinking can be taught within health professions schools as well as in undergraduate premed programs and the health humanities. Typically, students in medicine, nursing, pharmacy, and other health professions programs become stuck in passive-learning environments that focus on memorization and rely on assessment conducted via multiple-choice questions. To avoid sitting in large lecture halls and listening to 60-minute PowerPoint lectures by their professors, many students choose to watch recorded lectures on their computers—often at 1.5x speed! Traditional health sciences curricula have done a good job of producing highly specialized technicians. But they rarely inspire creativity and imaginative ideas.

The pedagogy for health design thinking is built on studio-based learning. This learning model is fundamental for architecture, industrial design, graphic design, and creative disciplines. Studios allow students to develop creative thinking, oral and visual presentation skills, and the ability to work in teams. The active learning environment of the studio is open-ended and informal but no less rigorous than passive, classroom-based teaching.

Courses in health design thinking help students master the skills of observing, imagining, and making. Such a curriculum does not seek to turn future doctors and nurses into designers. A design mindset can help learners acquire fresh insights and activate their creative agency. The future of health care needs the next generation of clinicians and leaders to be able not only to find the right answers but also to search for the right questions.

Courses in health design thinking are built around a specific challenge or issue in health care. These challenges can range from improving the patient experience in a busy urban outpatient primary clinic to increasing access to psychiatric services in a rural area. The length of a course can range from a few weeks to multiple semesters.

In a studio-based learning model, learners identify real-world problems in health care and develop solutions through a hands-on creative process. Students explore and apply the methods of health design thinking in a way that's not possible in a traditional classroom. In the most vital educational environments, students learn by doing.

See one, do one, teach one.

A health design thinking course centers on a design project where teams design a product, service, or space in response to a specific challenge.

Divide students into teams of 3–6 people. Each team develops its own project. Working in a team helps students acquire skills of managing, collaborating, and resolving conflict. The delivery of health care is team based; we don't work in isolation.

Introduce concepts through hands-on tutorials, mini-workshops, and engagement with design practitioners and stakeholders. Avoid giving long PowerPoint presentations.

Use the Method chapters in this book to introduce the principles of Health Design Thinking during active, hands-on sessions.

Reinforce design principles with rapid-fire team activities that include sketching, presenting, and making as well as interviewing and observing.

Produce a rhythm of "teach-do-debrief." Debrief often with your teams. Ask, "What went well?" or "What could have gone better?"

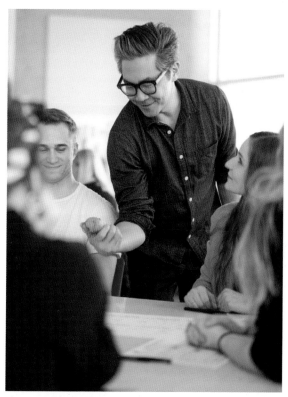

Photo: David Campbell

THE STUDIO CRITIQUE Multiple-choice exams cannot accurately assess learners in Health Design Thinking courses. If possible, avoid using them and make these courses pass/fail. The design critique or "crit" is the best vehicle for assessment. Crits help designers build confidence by sharing their work, accepting feedback, and revising ideas.

Schedule routine crits throughout a course. Invite colleagues and the general public to participate. If a team is designing a mobile app to help patients with diabetes eat healthier, be sure to include people living with diabetes in the design process. Clinicians, caregivers, and hospital adminstrators could also be stakeholders.

CREATIVE COLLABORATORS You don't need to be a designer to run a Health Design Thinking course. In fact, it is unlikely that you will find a design educator at your health system or medical school. If you are a clinician, your role will be to introduce real-world challenges in the health care environment to the course. Search for designers and others to act as workshop facilitators or critiquers for project reviews. Here are some of the professionals we have invited to co-teach classes: architects, graphic designers, industrial designers, visual artists, service designers, UX/UI designers, medical device engineers, app developers, journalists, and actors.

START SMALL Introducing health design thinking into your clinic, hospital, or university might seem like a daunting task. But there are many points of entry for a human-centered design approach in medicine. Start by doing. If you lack funding to launch a full-length course, for example, prototype your concept through a pop-up event. Host an informal meetup or deliver a design workshop that invites anyone interested in the topic. These pop-ups may stir student interest, get buy-in from administrators, and attract collaborators. If you work in a health care system, try applying design methods to a clinical challenge. Running a workshop with stakeholders, storyboarding solutions to problems, or creating a journey map centered on a patient experience may drive institutional support to fund a health design project and inspire others to join you.

Look beyond your own domain of expertise for help. A physician with a busy clinical practice may not have the time needed to learn how to create and implement design solutions. Try collaborating with designers from universities or firms that have an interest in health.

A short workshop or even a yearlong course won't result in a market-ready product or a systemic change in the health care system. But any experience with design can challenge people's assumptions about medicine.

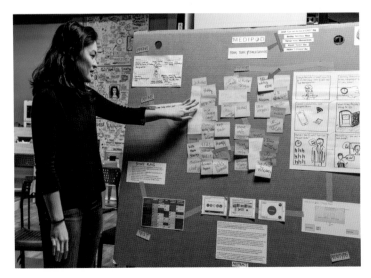

PRESENTATION SKILLS During critiques, team members restate the problem they are attempting to solve and explain their solution through storytelling. Presentations can take the form of slide decks, project visualization boards, and prototype demonstrations.

Create your own health design challenges

PROMPT	TOPICS AND ACTIVITIES
PATIENT EXPERIENCE *Put yourself in the shoes of a patient and redesign a health care service or experience.*	Pick up a medication at a pharmacy. Check in as a new patient in a doctor's office. Get blood drawn at a lab. Schedule an appointment with a specialist. Get a chest X-ray. Eat food from a hospital menu. Fill out an insurance form. Sign up for a patient portal. Read through a patient discharge summary. Discuss code status with a clinician. Talk to a caregiver. Ask an insurance representative to explain a bill. Imagine being a child getting an MRI or a CT scan.
FIELD OBSERVATION *Look beyond your own area of expertise and discover the pain points experienced by others.*	Nurse Physician Receptionist Pharmacist Phlebotomist Lab technician Clinical supervisor Administrator Patient Caregiver Medical biller
INCLUSIVE DESIGN *Look through the eyes of people living with disabilities or chronic conditions that limit mobility. Observe or listen to the challenges that they face on a daily basis.*	Curbs and sidewalks Doorknobs Light switches Steps Showers Meals Public transportation
WAYFINDING *Improve the signage and navigation within health care facilities.*	Find the exit of an emergency department. Walk from the parking lot to an inpatient room. Locate the hospital cafeteria. Use a wheelchair and find an accessible restroom. Search for the surgical waiting room. Locate a phone-charging station. Find a place to rest.
IMPROVE THE EHR *Search for ways to improve the EHR system.*	Find the image of an EKG in a patient chart. Reconcile an outpatient medication history. Update a patient's drug allergies. Order an imaging study. Access the most recent discharge summary. Find the results for the most recent urine culture.

IMAGINE THE FUTURE OF . . . *Imagine what health care will be like* *in fifty years.*	Hospitals Clinics Surgeries End-of-life care Diabetes EHR Telehealth
MAPPING JOURNEYS *Show others the steps that a user takes* *during a health care service.*	Being hospitalized Visiting an ER Delivering a baby Having a routine colonoscopy Getting hemodialysis Having radiation therapy
RETHINKING PRODUCTS *Create a low-fidelity prototype for a* *redesigned medical device or product.*	Patient gown IV catheter Cardiac monitor Hospital bed Prescription bottle Surgical instrument
CHALLENGING THE STATUS QUO *Pick something routinely done in health* *care that may not be necessary. Create an* *alternate scenario.*	Frequently taking vital signs on stable patients Scheduling frequent follow-up visits with your doctor Sitting in a waiting room Scheduling an annual physical exam Conducting morning lab tests on hospitalized patients Scheduling medical appointments by phone
FINDING ANALOGOUS INSPIRATION *Get a fresh perspective on improving a* *product or service by looking at industries* *outside of health care.*	Airbnb Amazon Prime Your favorite restaurant Netflix Four Seasons hotel Airline industry
DESIGNING SPACE *Redesign a physical space in a health* *care facility.*	Clinic Operating room Nursing workstation Reception area Exam room Hospital patient room Postoperative recovery room Family waiting area
DESIGNING PROCESS *Pick a hospital protocol, clinical* *pathway, or process and make it* *simpler.*	Preoperative clearance Hospital discharge Inpatient admission Hospital transfer Patient handoff Sepsis protocol Acute stroke pathway

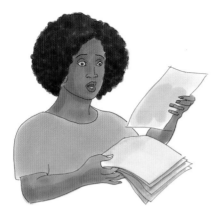

Discharge instructions are supposed to help patients and caregivers understand how to manage their health after leaving the hospital. Alas, the experience is often an overwhelming data dump. How could you change this process? Whom should you interview to learn more about the problem?

EXTREME USERS
Gain inspiration by observing and engaging with individuals or populations who fall outside the majority of users of a health care service.

Non-English speaking
Food insecure
Transgender
Immigrant
Unstable housing
Disabled
Uninsured
Refugee
Elderly
Medical professional/expert

ROLE PLAYING
Understand the experience of clinicians by acting out real-life scenarios.

Navigate a difficult patient encounter.
Experience multiple disruptions in a task.
Call another hospital for medical records.
Deliver bad news to a patient.
Call an insurance company to preauthorize test.
Find time for self-care (eating food, using a restroom, etc.) during a busy shift.
Run behind schedule during an outpatient clinic.

SOCIAL DETERMINANTS OF HEALTH
Understand the nonmedical factors that impact health.

Create a healthy meal for less than $3.
Take public transit from a poor zip code to a hospital.
Purchase groceries in a food desert.
Find safe play areas in a low-income neighborhood.
Visit a homeless shelter.
Visit a patient whose race/ethnicity differs from yours.
Engage with local community-based organizations.

DIGITAL HEALTH
Prototype a mobile health app that improves lives of patients.

Communicating with clinicians
Conducting medical billing
Searching for clinical trials
Developing patient communities
Promoting medication adherence
Finding specialists
Addressing mental health
Offering behavioral therapy
Providing discharge instructions

3D Printing

The applications of 3D printing in health care extend far beyond customizing hip implants for patients or transplanting 3D-printed organs. With desktop 3D printers and open-source software, novices can print anatomical models for surgical planning, build high-fidelity prototypes for new medical devices, and design bespoke tools for biomedical research.

3D anatomical models are superior to flat, 2D, computerized images of computerized tomography (CT) or magnetic resonance imaging (MRI) scans for understanding human anatomy. Holding a physical, patient-specific anatomical model in your hands provides both surgeon and patient with a richness of spatial data that is missing from CT or MRI scans. 3D printing can decrease operating room times, give surgeons better spatial data for planning cases, and improve patient communication.

A multidisciplinary team composed of obstetrician-gynecologists, radiologists, medical students, and health design faculty at Thomas Jefferson University designed and 3D-printed a model of the uterus of a patient who had fibroids to decrease the risk of complications during her planned cesarean delivery. If a surgeon accidentally makes an incision into a fibroid, the resulting blood loss can be significant. To give the mother and her baby the best chance for a successful operation, the team used the 3D model to plan the case and brought the model to the operating room for real-time guidance.

Scientists and researchers require highly specific laboratory tools to conduct their research. 3D printing is being used by scientists to build customized tools and replacement parts for lab equipment. 3D printing has been used to create scaffolding structures for growing uniformly seeded cells, and a microfluidic device that is used to apply fluid sheer stress to osteoblast cells. This ability to prototype tools can save research labs thousand of dollars.

3D printing puts precision manufacturing in the hands of a wide range of users—from clinicians to biomedical researchers—and opens up the possibility for medical educators and students to develop new training tools. As a technique for health design thinking, 3D printing enables new possibilities for visualizing and prototyping.

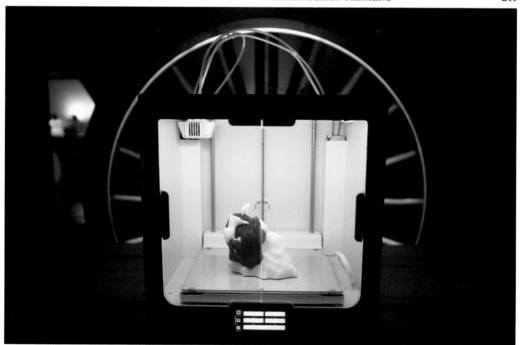

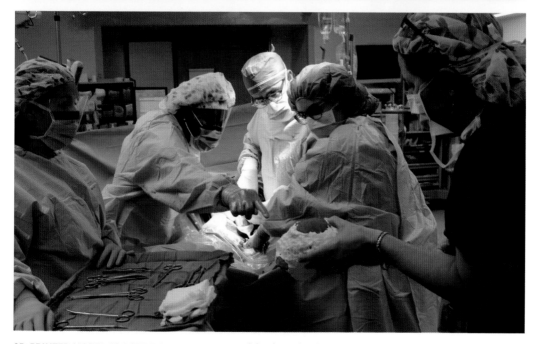

3D-PRINTED MODEL FOR SURGICAL PLANNING Models of a patient's placenta and uterus helped the surgical team avoid accidentally incising fibroid tumors during a cesarean delivery.

ANATOMICAL MODELS FOR TRAINING 3D models are invaluable training tools for physicians. For example, drilling into the temporal bone is one of the most common procedures in otolaryngology. Surgical residents must practice this procedure before performing on patients, because of the risk of complications. Drilling in the wrong area by just a few millimeters can result in venous bleeding, facial nerve paralysis, and permanent hearing loss. Currently, training for this procedure requires that temporal bones be harvested from cadavers; these bones are expensive and in limited supply. 3D-printed temporal bones offer a low-cost alternative that mimics the look and feel of real cadaveric bone.

Simulation-based learning allows clinicians to hone their procedural skills without harming patients. Medical training simulators are widely available commercially but are extremely expensive. 3D printing allows for educators in health professional schools to design and build their own low-cost simulators.

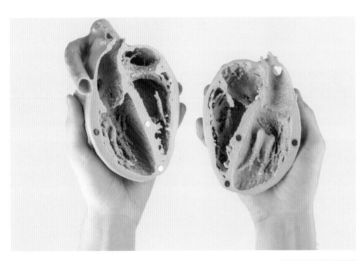

MODELING THE HEART
Someone who will be conducting cardiac ultrasounds needs to understand the heart—no easy task. 3D heart models were created to train physicians to perform echocardiograms. These models are sliced into specific planes that match the standard views of an echocardiogram. It's easier for learners to obtain the correct image on an ultrasound if they can match it to a physical model of the heart.

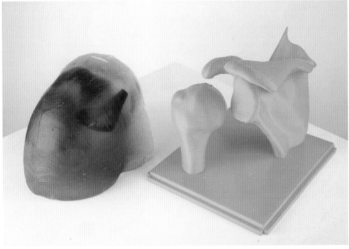

TRAINING SIMULATORS
A 3D-printed shoulder joint is used for simulating the delivery of ultrasound-guided shoulder injections. The shoulder joint (right) is placed inside a molded mass of gelatin (left). The bones are visualized through the gelatin by an ultrasound machine.

Photos: David Campbell

Setting up a 3D printing lab

Explore open-source software to convert CT and MRI scans into 3D-print-ready files.

Purchase a low-cost desktop 3D printer instead of a high-end industrial 3D printer.

Practice printing open-source anatomical models from the NIH 3D Print Exchange.

Find partners—radiologists, surgeons, students—to identify clinical projects that will benefit from 3D printing.

Develop a plan to publish your findings in peer-reviewed journals or at conferences.

READ MORE → www.machinedesign.com/3d-printing/look-future-medical-3d-printing-part-1

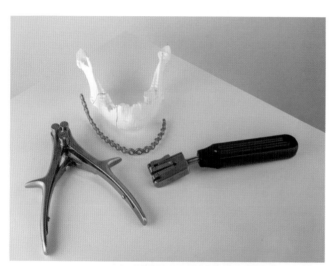

ANATOMICAL MODELS FOR SURGICAL PLANNING 3D printing has been used in surgical cases for patients with cancer that has invaded the jawbone. A model of the patient's bone is printed before surgery. The titanium plate used to stabilize the bone can be bent to match the patient's anatomy prior to surgery. This pre-bent plate reduces the time needed to perform this laborious task in the operating room. Photos: David Campbell (top) and Robert Pugliese (bottom)

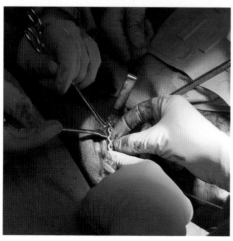

Designing Medical Devices

Health care is full of poorly designed devices and products. Anyone who sets foot in a clinical setting has seen this problem in action, from incessantly beeping monitors to user-unfriendly epinephrine autoinjector pens. Errors associated with medical devices are costly and cause harm to thousands of people each year. Patients, nurses, doctors, and caregivers are well positioned to develop concepts for better products but often lack the know-how to bring ideas to life.

Health design thinking empowers stakeholders to create new medical devices and improve the functionality of existing ones. You don't need to be an engineer to invent better products. A common misconception is that new medical devices must be high tech, complex, and expensive. The health care industry is full of opportunities that require simple interventions or improvements. If problems are solved well, their solutions can have a substantial, measurable impact on a systemic scale.

Nonetheless, translating an idea for a new device into an FDA-approved, commercially viable product is a herculean task. There is no recipe for simplifying this process. However, starting the process journey by asking good questions and applying design principles can set development in the right direction. The design principles embodied by a product will help determine whether clinicians will desire to use or prescribe the device, whether hospital administrators will purchase it, and whether patients will benefit from its use.

Questions to ask about a product idea

How has this problem been addressed before?

What is the fundamental problem you are trying to solve?

Who are the users, the consumers, and the purchasers?

What value will the solution provide to the user, the consumer, and the purchaser?

What are the foreseen obstacles and opportunities?

How will I validate this idea?

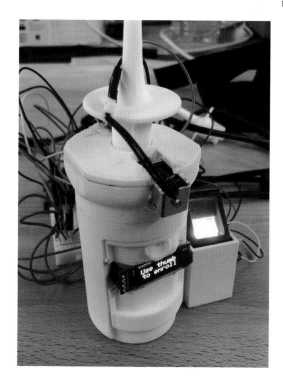

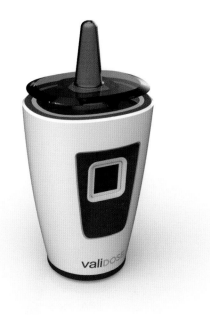

SUBSTANCE CONTROL Validose, an intranasal drug delivery device, solves the problem of delivering esketamine (a form of ketamine) to patients with treatment-resistant depression. The design had to address the challenges of dosing accurately, ensuring security, preventing abuse, and integrating with existing treatment workflows. To use Validose, a physician inputs the desired dosage and frequency and patients use their fingerprint to unlock the device and dispense medication. Design: 10xBeta

Design principles for product development

Intuitive to use

Improves the efficiency of existing workflows

Consistent and reliable performance

Creates value for all stakeholders

Sustainability: sterilizable, reusable, reduces waste

ADLER DESIGN Founded by Deborah Adler, this multidisciplinary studio has pioneered design solutions for diverse projects ranging from clearer medication labels on prescription bottles to redesigned packaging for foley catheters.

ARIADNE LABs This joint innovation center of Brigham and Women's Hospital and the Harvard T.H. Chan School of Public Health creates programs and projects rooted in rigorous scientific methodology and best practices to improve health systems and patient lives.

THE BETTER LAB A research program within the University of California, San Francisco's Zuckerberg San Francisco General Hospital uses design to study and fix health care challenges.

CARE+WEAR This company incorporates fashion and design to create products, such as PICC line covers and mobility gloves, that improve patient comfort and satisfaction.

CENTER FOR SOCIAL DESIGN, Maryland Institute College of Art (MICA). The Center demonstrates design's role in advancing equity and social justice and works to prepare the next generation of creative changemakers.

THE CENTER FOR UNIVERSAL DESIGN Founded in 1989 at North Carolina State University College of Design, this research center is dedicated to universal design. At the time of of this publishing, the Center is unstaffed because of lack of funding; however, the website is an important repository of principles and resources.

COOPER HEWITT, SMITHSONIAN DESIGN MUSEUM The only museum in the U.S. dedicated to historical and contemporary design, Cooper Hewitt produces lectures, workshops, exhibitions, publications, and curricula on human-centered design, inclusive design, design for social justice, and other areas of design theory and practice.

DALBERG DESIGN This global design and innovation practice has partnered with USAID and the Bill & Melinda Gates Foundation on global health projects, from redesigning personal protective equipment for healthcare workers to building design resources for global health practitioners.

DESIGN COUNCIL Established in 1944, the Design Council acts as the U.K. government's advisor on design. It uses design as a strategic tool to tackle societal challenges, drive economic growth and innovation, and improve the quality of the built environment.

DESIGN FOR HEALTH This invaluable collection of methods and case studies translates published evidence into tools for health practitioners. The aim is to strengthen demand for design within the global health community.

DESIGN INSTITUTE FOR HEALTH A collaboration between Dell Medical School and the College of Fine Arts at the University of Texas at Austin, the Institute applies design thinking to complex challenges in health care.

DESIGN THINKING FOR HEALTH This online platform (designthinkingforhealth.org) highlights the work of nurse innovators in the U.S. and provides resources focused on design thinking.

GOINVO This Boston-based digital design studio focuses on better health access and outcomes through design. Working exclusively in the health care space, GoInvo designs products and services for health systems, companies, and governmental agencies.

GOOD HEALTH DESIGN Based in New Zealand, this team of transdisciplinary researchers at Auckland University of Technology's School of Art + Design uses design to improve the health and well-being of communities.

GREATER GOOD STUDIO Based in Chicago, this strategic design firm focuses on advancing equity by creating human-centered programs, building tools and experiences, and teaching design methods to changemakers.

HEALTH DESIGN LAB, EMILY CARR UNIVERSITY At this research and design center in Vancouver, Canada, design faculty and students work collaboratively on projects that address complex challenges in health and health care.

HEALTH DESIGN LAB, JEFFERSON UNIVERSITY Founded in 2016, the Health Design Lab is part of the Sidney Kimmel Medical College at Thomas Jefferson University in Philadelphia. The Health Design Lab creates workshops, courses, and curricula for medical students, clinicians, patients, and members of the health care industry.

HEALTHCARE HUMAN FACTORS Based in Toronto General Hospital, this team of human factors professionals, designers, engineers, psychologists, and researchers works to make health care safer.

HEALTHCARE INNOVATION COLLABORATORY Located in the University of Vermont Health Network, this design and innovation lab codesigns with patients, providers, staff, and community members to improve experiences for patients and employees.

HELIX CENTRE Based in London, the Centre is an interdisciplinary group of designers, technologists, clinicians, and researchers that uses human-centered design to understand problems in health care and develop clinically evaluated solutions.

IBM DESIGN A global company with more than 2,000 designers, IBM published resources on its framework, called Enterprise Design Thinking. Learn more about IBM's principles and approach at → www.ibm.com/design/thinking/.

THE IDEA CENTER (Center for Inclusive Design and Environmental Access) The IDeA Center is dedicated to making environments and products safer, more usable, and healthier in response to the needs of diverse populations. The IDeA Center's website features numerous case studies and documents related to inclusive design, often called "universal design" or "design for all."

IDEO From designing the first manufacturable mouse for Apple to advancing the practice of human-centered design, IDEO has long been at the forefront of creating change through design and disseminating design methodologies.

IDEO.ORG This not-for-profit organization is an offshoot of the global design consultancy IDEO. Design Kit is an online learning platform that explains the mindsets and methods of human-centered design and provides a platform for a global innovation community.

KAISER PERMANENTE DESIGN CONSULTANCY This consultancy designs solutions for health care challenges across Kaiser Permanente, one of the largest not-for-profit health insurers in the U.S.

KIERANTIMBERLAKE This architecture firm is committed to integrating research and design. It has received numerous design awards and recognitions, including the Cooper Hewitt National Design Award for Architecture (2010).

MAKERHEALTH SPACE AT THE UNIVERSITY OF TEXAS MEDICAL BRANCH This first makerspace in a hospital is a place for the community to design, build, and prototype.

MASS DESIGN GROUP MASS, a nonprofit architecture firm, has designed hospitals and facilities in Rwanda, Haiti, Malawi, and the Democratic Republic of Congo. The group received the Cooper Hewitt National Design Award for Architecture (2017).

MAYO CLINIC CENTER FOR INNOVATION The Center brings designers and physicians together to apply design thinking to transform the experience and delivery of health and health care in a large system that treats over one million patients per year.

MEDICAL FUTURES LAB AT RICE UNIVERSITY This multidisciplinary collaborative learning lab seeks to study and understand the intersection of medicine and technology. The MFL includes a focus on undergraduate education.

MIT LITTLE DEVICES LAB The Lab explores the design, invention, and policy spaces for DIY health technologies around the world.

NOWPOW This knowledge utility company helps underserved communities by providing people with the vital information they need to stay well and live long.

NG TENG FONG CENTRE FOR HEALTHCARE INNOVATION Based in Singapore, the Centre uses design-based pedagogy to train health care professionals via interactive learning, teaching, and research.

OMADA HEALTH One of the pioneering companies in digital behavioral medicine, Omada Health uses online programs to tackle the growing epidemic of type 2 diabetes, heart disease, and obesity.

OPENLAB Located at the University Health Network in Toronto, OpenLab is dedicated to finding creative solutions that transform the way health care is delivered and experienced.

OPEN STYLE LAB This nonprofit organization comprises a team of designers, engineers, and occupational therapists who create functional wearable solutions for people of all abilities without compromising on style. OSL won the 2019 National Design Award for an Emerging Designer.

PATIENT REVOLUTION This nonprofit organization develops tools, programs, and resources that help patients, caregivers, communities, and clinicians work toward health care that is careful and kind. Resources can be found at → patientrevolution.org.

PEARSONLLOYD This London-based design consultancy works across various sectors, including aviation, workplace, urban design, and health care.

PICTAL HEALTH Led by Katie McCurdy, a designer and a patient with an autoimmune condition, Pictal Health helps patients visually communicate their health histories.

PILLPACK A full-service online pharmacy, Pillpack has redesigned the pharmacy experience for patients.

STANFORD D.SCHOOL Founded in 2004, the d.school is a place where people from diverse disciplines and fields of study use design to develop their own creative potential.

STANFORD MEDICINE X Led by Dr. Larry Chu, this program focuses on patient-centered innovation and explores the intersection of emerging technology and medicine.

SUTTER HEALTH DESIGN & INNOVATION This team, based in Sutter Health's twenty-four-hospital network in Northern California, looks across the health care journey for opportunities to improve care before, during, and after the patient visit.

WELLCOME COLLECTION This free museum and library in London invites people to reflect on the rich connections among science, medicine, life, and art. The Wellcome Collection offers exhibitions, collections, live programming, publishing, and online resources related to health, medicine, and the humanities.

HUMAN-CENTERED DESIGN

Brown, Tim. *Change by Design: How Design Thinking Transforms Organizations and Inspires Innovation.* New York: Harper Business, 2012.

Guffey, Elizabeth. *Designing Disability: Symbols, Space, Society.* London: Bloomsbury, 2018.

Jones, Peter. *Design for Care: Innovating Healthcare Experience.* New York: Rosenfeld Media, 2013.

Holmes, Kat. *Mismatch: How Inclusion Shapes Design.* Cambridge: MIT Press, 2018.

Löwgren, Jonas, and Bo Reimer. *Collaborative Media, Production, Consumption, and Design Interventions.* Cambridge: MIT Press, 2013.

Norman, Don. *The Design of Everyday Things: Revised and Expanded Edition.* New York: Basic Books, 2013.

Pullen, Graham. *Design Meets Disability.* Cambridge: MIT Press, 2009.

Sanders, Elizabeth B.-N., and Pieter Jan Stappers. *Convivial Toolbox: Generative Research for the Front End of Design.* Amsterdam: BIS, 2012.

Schrank, Sarah, and Didem Ekici, eds. *Healing Spaces, Modern Architecture, and the Body.* London: Routledge, 2017.

Stickdorn, Marc. *This Is Service Design Thinking: Basics, Tools, Cases.* Hoboken, NJ: Wiley, 2012.

Tsekleves, Emmanuel and Rachel Cooper. *Design for Health.* London: Routledge, 2017.

Williamson, Bess. *Accessible America: A History of Disability and Design.* New York: New York University Press, 2019.

ONLINE READING

The Business Value of Design. → www.mckinsey.com/business-functions/mckinsey-design/our-insights/the-business-value-of-design

The Field Guide to Human-Centered Design (IDEO). → www.designkit.org/resources

Health Care Providers Can Use Design Thinking to Improve Patient Experiences. → hbr.org/2017/08/health-care-providers-can-use-design-thinking-to-improve-patient-experiences

Making Design Thinking a Part of Medical Education. → catalyst.nejm.org/making-design-thinking-part-medical-education/

The Total Economic Impact™ Of IBM's Design Thinking Practice. → www.ibm.com/design/thinking/static/media/Enterprise-Design-Thinking-Report.8ab1e9e1.pdf

PEER-REVIEWED JOURNAL ARTICLES

Altman, Myra, Huang, Terry T. K., and Breland, Jessica Y. "Design Thinking in Health Care." *Preventing Chronic Disease* 15, no. 9 (2020): E117.

Asch, David A. et al. "Insourcing Health Care Innovation." *The New England Journal of Medicine* 370, no. 19 (2014): 1775–7.

Brown, Tim, and Wyatt, Jocelyn. "Design Thinking for Social Innovation." *Stanford Social Innovation Review* 8, no. 1 (Winter 2010): 31–35.

Donetto, Sarah et al. "Experience-Based Codesign and Healthcare Improvement: Realizing Participatory Design in the Public Sector." *The Design Journal*, 18, no. 2 (2015): 227–48.

Eberhart, A. et al. "Using a Human-Centered Design Approach for Collaborative Decision-Making in Pediatric Asthma Care." *Public Health* 170 (2019): 129–32.

Gottlieb, Michael et al. "Applying Design Thinking Principles to Curricular Development in Medical Education." *AEM Education and Training* 1, no. 1 (2017): 21–26.

Martin, Molly A. et al. "Engaging End-Users in Intervention Research Study Design." *Journal of Asthma* 55, no. 5 (2018): 483–91.

Matheson, Gordon O. et al. "Leveraging Human-Centered Design in Chronic Disease Prevention." *American Journal of Preventive Medicine* 48, no. 4 (2015): 472–79.

Robert, Glenn et al. "Patients and Staff as Codesigners of Healthcare Services." *BMJ : British Medical Journal* 350 (2015): g7714.

Roberts, Jess P. et al. "A Design Thinking Framework for Healthcare Management and Innovation." *Healthcare* 4, no. 1 (2016): 11–14.

Vechakul, Jessica et al. "Human-Centered Design as an Approach for Place-Based Innovation in Public Health: A Case Study from Oakland, California." *Maternal and Child Health Journal* 19, no. 12 (2015): 2552–9.

HEALTH AND THE MEDICAL INDUSTRY

Ehrenreich, Barbara. *Natural Causes: An Epidemic of Wellness, the Certainty of Dying, and Killing Ourselves to Live Longer.* New York: Twelve, 2018.

Topol, Eric. *The Patient Will See You Now: The Future of Medicine Is in Your Hands.* New York: Basic Books, 2016.

Wachter, Robert. *The Digital Doctor: Hope, Hype, and Harm at the Dawn of Medicine's Computer Age.* New York: McGraw-Hill, 2017.

Trying to give thanks to all the amazing humans who have contributed to this book is a herculean task. First, I want to honor the thousands of patients that I have treated in emergency departments in Philadelphia. Their stories and experiences touch every page of this book.

Ellen Lupton is my design hero. When I first read her books, I immediately knew that we needed a book like hers for health care. I thank Ellen for her incredible generosity and constant encouragement, and for letting me into her world of writing about design. Creating this book with Ellen has given me fresh insight and deeper empathy. Although Ellen is not a physician, her creative approach to solving problems and explaining concepts can help all of us who serve the needs of patients.

Pamela Horn's enthusiasm for the book inspired me, and her keen oversight made the content stronger. Jennifer Tobias created beautiful illustrations that capture the art and science of medicine. Caroline Baumann, Director of Cooper Hewitt, Smithsonian Design Museum, provided the ideal platform to publish my first book.

I am indebted to my extraordinary team at the Health Design Lab at Thomas Jefferson University: Robert Pugliese, Andrea Landau, Geoffrey Hayden, Kristy Shine, Erik Backlund, and Matthew Fields. Rob cofounded the Health Design Lab with me, and every day he pours his talent into bringing human-centered design into the health care space. Thanks also to the medical students who choose to study health design thinking with us. They are the true brains of our operation.

This book would not have been possible without the unwavering support of Mark Tykocinski and Stephen Klasko, visionary leaders in medical education and health care. Special thanks to the rest of my Jefferson family: Theodore Christopher, Bernard Lopez, Donna Gentile O'Donnell, Rose Ritts, Emergency Medicine faculty and residents, and the staff and nurses with whom I work in the ER.

Lastly, I am indebted to Mindy, Naomi, and Nolan. I love you guys.

— Bon Ku, MD

Creating this book with Bon Ku has been a thrilling opportunity to grow and learn. Bon's work combines empirical rigor with kindness, creativity, and the belief that everyone on Earth deserves quality health care. I gained fresh insight from Bon's outstanding colleagues, including Serene Chen, Geoffrey Hayden, Robert S. Pugliese, and Kristy Shine.

Deep gratitude goes to my longtime friend and collaborator Jennifer Tobias. In addition to creating dozens of illustrations for this book, she developed an astonishing number of cover designs, which Bon shared for comment with clinicians at Thomas Jefferson University. Some covers were pronounced dead on arrival while others were sent back for radical surgery and rehab. We finally found a viable heartbeat with the friendly stethoscope that graces the cover of this book. (Much thanks to Ann Sunwoo for tweaking the typography.)

I owe endless thanks to Pamela Horn, Cooper Hewitt's Director of Cross-Platform Publishing, for her extraordinary ability to bring content to the public— and for her loving and supportive friendship. From the first meeting we convened with Bon in Cooper Hewitt's garden, Pam saw what this book could be, and she used her energy and talent to make it happen. I am grateful to Caroline Baumann, Director of Cooper Hewitt, National Design Museum, and Curatorial Director Cara McCarty, for allowing me to create this book, and to Matthew Kennedy, Cross-Platform Publishing Associate, for his editorial craft.

In addition to my role at Cooper Hewitt, Smithsonian Design Museum, I am on the faculty at MICA (Maryland Institute College of Art). This book includes outstanding contributions from my colleagues in MICA's Center for Social Design; special thanks go to Ashley K. Eberhart, Becky Slogeris, and Mike Weikert.

None of my books would happen without my family. Many thanks to my parents, Mary Jane Lupton, Ken Baldwin, William Lupton, and Lauren Carter; to my sister, Julia Reinhard Lupton; to my children, Jay and Ruby Miller; to my talented husband, Abbott Miller; to Jack, Kevin, and the fabulous Miller sisters; and to my MICA family, Jennifer Cole Phillips and Brockett Horne.

— Ellen Lupton

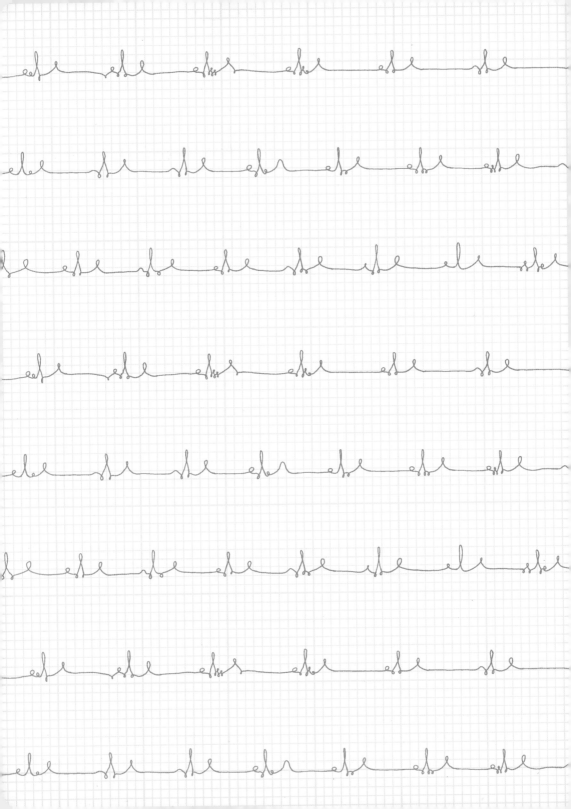